W9-BOP-405

"An honest, warm, and distinctively Christian approach to overcoming nicotine addiction. Highly recommended."

Dr. David G. Myers
Professor of Psychology
Hope College, Holland, Michigan

"I highly recommend the program this book describes to anyone who is ready to quit smoking. It is a giant step toward taking responsibility for ourselves and our health."

Suzanne Taylor
Now a nonsmoker, thanks to the
Stop-smoking Clinic, June 1985

"The stop-smoking program outlined in this book meets a clear need. Nonsmokers have better attendance records, less lost time, and generally better health. Business should support the elimination of smoking as a major goal for the good of all."

L. L. Bratschie
President
Executive Resources International

Living Without Smoking

How to Survive When You're Ready to Quit

Marilyn Vander Veen
John W. Stewart
Susie Heritage

AUGSBURG • MINNEAPOLIS

LIVING WITHOUT SMOKING
How to Survive When You're Ready to Quit

Copyright © 1989 Augsburg Fortress

All rights reserved. Except for brief quotations in critical articles or reviews, no part of this book may be reproduced in any manner without prior written permission from the publisher. Write to: Permissions, Augsburg Fortress, 426 S. Fifth St., Box 1209, Minneapolis MN 55440.

Scripture quotations unless otherwise noted are from the Holy Bible: New International Version. Copyright 1978 by the New York International Bible Society. Used by permission of Zondervan Bible Publishers.

Cover design: Koechel/Peterson Design

Library of Congress Cataloging-in-Publication Data

Vander Veen, Marilyn, 1933–
    Living without smoking : how to survive when you're ready to
      quit
  / Marilyn Vander Veen, John W. Stewart, and Susie Heritage.
      p.   cm.
    Bibliography: p.
    ISBN 0-8066-2413-2
    1. Smoking.   2. Cigarette habit.   3. Cigarette habit—Treatment.
I. Stewart, John W., 1933–   . II: Heritage, Susie, 1944–   .
III. Title.
HV5733.V33   1989
616.86'506—dc20   89-31948
                                    CIP

Manufactured in the U.S.A.   AF 9-2413

1 2 3 4 5 6 7 8 9 0 1 2 3 4 5 6 7 8 9

Contents

Preface

O ne brilliant fall afternoon I received a call from Marilyn Vander Veen, an elder in the congregation I serve. "I'm in serious trouble," she said. "I just returned from seeing my doctor. He says that I am in the early stages of emphysema. It is so severe and so enveloping that unless I quit smoking immediately my life will be threatened." She paused, choking back tears. "I am very frightened and I don't know what to do or where to turn. Can you—or God—or somebody tell me how to quit?" she sobbed softly.

I didn't know where to begin or what to say. I too was struggling with my own addiction to pipe smoking. On and off, I had puffed away since seminary days. The more intense and stressful my pastoral duties, the more pipe smoke I made. Ill-disguised coughs, sore throats, and little burn holes in my trousers were more than telltale indications that I was only a little different from Marilyn. Embarrassed by my own pathetic witness and sensing that her pain was to become, inevitably, mine also, I said, "Let's both quit. Now! I'll help you, if you'll help me."

I blurted out, half by inspiration, half in panic, "Let's get some smokers together and go on a retreat. We'll try to learn together how to quit. And if we can learn, maybe we can help others to quit, too." I hardly appreciated what came out of my own mouth. I genuinely wanted to help her—she was deeply threatened and frightened—but I wasn't at all sure of to what I had obligated myself.

Thirteen people from various walks of life signed up for that first retreat. Imagine living with 13 people, all of them trying to quit smoking! One getting up at four o'clock in the morning to jog, another pacing and unable to sleep, one sulking in a corner, and all talking about how much they wanted to smoke. What began to emerge, however, was a beginning for a different pattern of living with healthier substitutes for smoking. The retreat weekend was a success and we began planning for another.

Out of that impromptu covenant I had made with Marilyn, a citywide, lay-led, inexpensive, spiritually grounded, grass roots ministry to help others quit the smoking habit was developed. Under Marilyn's leadership, the emerging team of Christian laypeople from our church, Westminster Presbyterian, and our neighboring church, Eastminster Presbyterian, refined their program and retreats. Soon hospitals, major manufacturing companies, and other congregations sought our services. Today, 10 years later, the demand for us to share our experience and expertise exceeds our capacities to fill all outside requests.

From the very beginning we emphasized that our program is a Christian-based ministry. We really believe that God wants wholeness for all persons and that God is "alive and well" and mightily at work to empower persons who are otherwise powerless to quit destructive habits. The biblical word for salvation is derived from a family of words related to health and wholeness. The care of bodies is no less a Christian responsibility than the care of souls. Further, we believe this ministry to be an appropriate expression of a Christian congregation. It is more than fulfilling the current adage to "find a need and fill it." Rather, this ministry has emerged as an expression of the gospel, a model in lay-equipped ministries, and an authentic service to others who desperately—or even *not* so desperately—want to quit smoking. Time has tested our efforts and many people have learned how to quit smoking through this particular experiment in congregation-based ministry.

Are you a smoker? Do you want to quit? Are you reading this book in hopes of finding a way of giving up the habit? Well, we would like to share with you what we have learned these last 10 years. We would like to walk you through the basics of the program that has helped us kick the nicotine habit. We hope that it will help motivate *you* to give up smoking as well.

Our hope and prayer is that you will work through this book and will prayerfully and diligently apply its principles to your life. You can do it! Thousands of people quit smoking each year. For most of those people, giving up cigarettes is one of the most difficult—perhaps *the* most difficult—things they have ever done. But it can be done! The stop-smoking program which was the impetus for this book reflects a 40 percent success rate among its participants. Most programs say that about one-third of the participants succeed, and a U.S. Department of Health and Human Services statement reports that only 20 percent do (*Why People Smoke Cigarettes*, 1982).

You may use this book as a personal tool for quitting. With tremendous strength, determination, and the help of the Holy Spirit, you can become a nonsmoker on your own. But we strongly recommend that you become a part of a stop-smoking group. The sympathy, understanding, and support that you will find in such a group will be immeasurable. This program begins with your participation in a clinic or retreat and continues with ongoing support group meetings. You may wish to begin or encourage others to begin such a stop-smoking program in your church, community, business place, or local hospital. The Appendix of this book provides guidelines for setting up such a program. May God bless you in your efforts.

DR. JOHN W. STEWART

Acknowledgments

Stop-smoking Services has a list, 10 single-spaced pages long, of people and organizations who during the last 10 years have helped people give up their smoking habits. This is to acknowledge that effort and to say thank you.

Many thanks to Westminster and Eastminster Presbyterian Churches in Grand Rapids, Michigan, for sponsoring this ministry.

For those people who made the program possible and who keep it going, thank you. The names of that core group are scattered throughout the book.

When we were first collecting and organizing material for this book, our cheering section included Therese Campbell, Marsha Plafkin, and Susan Brondyk. Additional advice and inspiration came from Bob Vander Veen, Professors Sonja Stewart and David Myers, Bill Heritage, Dick and Marion Vander Veen, Peg Hertel, Steve Marshall, and Dan Van't Kerkhoff.

Marsha Hoffman, editor, has been indispensable in the formation of this book. If it weren't for her ability to sort and organize mass amounts of material, write some sections and rewrite others—and edit all—the book wouldn't have appeared in its present form. Thanks, Marsha, for making this all possible.

MARILYN VANDER VEEN
JACK STEWART
SUSIE HERITAGE

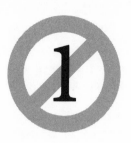

One Smoker's Story

Y ou're in the early stages of emphysema," my doctor said. "It is so severe, so enveloping, that unless you quit smoking *immediately*, you will not have long to live." Those death-sentence words echoed again and again as I drove home from the doctor's office. I knew the horror of emphysema, having watched my father-in-law, a heavy smoker, go through the agony of the disease, struggling for breath, and dying from both emphysema and lung cancer. Oh, yes, I knew the horror. And I knew that cigarette smoking is the chief cause of emphysema.

"I'll *have* to quit," I sobbed aloud, wiping away tears with the back of my hand. "But I can't, dear God, I just can't! I've tried before, and I just can't!" Tears poured down my face. I sensed God's nearness and I knew that somehow, some way I would—I *must*—quit smoking.

LOOKING BACK

My journey to stop smoking involved some difficult steps—steps that I forced myself to take one at a time.

13

My first step was to look back into my life, reflecting on how and why I smoked. Smoking didn't become a part of my life until I was in high school, and when it did, it was the "behind the barn smoke." "Why don't we try a cigarette?" the girls would dare at an overnight slumber party. The thrill was the lit cigarette between our lips and the knowledge that we were defying authority.

Determined to enjoy smoking and to perfect my smoking "skills," I began dating an older boy who smoked. I remember one date when I asked him to "park" so he could show me how to inhale cigarette smoke. To me, the secret to smoking was inhaling, and I was determined to learn to inhale—to swallow the smoke and then blow it back out. I lit the cigarette and swallowed the smoke, but instead of blowing it back out, I coughed until I thought I would vomit. My throat felt like it was on fire, but I was determined and I kept practicing until inhaling became routine.

Next, I began to concentrate on the proper way to hold the cigarette. My models were movie stars Lauren Bacall and Humphrey Bogart, whom I thought were incredibly sexy smokers. I practiced being slinky and sexy by the hour in front of the mirror until I felt I had the right look. I mastered the art of blowing smoke rings. "Sexy" and "smoke rings" seemed a good combination to me.

My mother detested smoking, whether it was cigar, cigarette, or pipe, and she was outrageously verbal about her feelings. When I would sneak a cigarette in the bathroom, blowing smoke out the open window, she would smell the smoke and lecture me about my "nasty habit." After high school graduation, I rebelled against parental authority and mother's fruitless lectures by moving out of my home. Freedom!

My newfound freedom and independence led me to a bigger smoking habit. When I had to make a decision, I sat, smoked, and thought out the situation. I was becoming psychologically, as well as physically, addicted to cigarette smoking. When I was lonely or afraid, the cigarette seemed to be a good friend. It quieted me down when I faced a crisis. It acted like a tranquilizer and gave me a euphoric feeling. Paradoxically, it sometimes acted as a stimulant and motivated me if I was tired and needed a lift.

The real reason I smoked, I told myself, was to stay slim. I'd lost 40 pounds since I'd left home and weighed a mere 98. When I smoked I didn't eat. I wanted to stay slim for my boyfriend, Bob. He drove a white convertible, had traveled extensively, and was a handsome, macho smoker. Bob and I eventually married, and we smoked together happily ever after—at least for 25 years! For me, smoking was thoroughly enjoyable. As enjoyable as it was though, I always knew deep down inside myself that it *was* a bad habit. Thus I attempted, from time to time, to give it up. But I didn't really want to. I began on these occasions to analyze my smoking habits and the games I played with my cigarette.

Why did I smoke?

Reflecting on my life began to give me clues about why I smoked. I realized that smoking meant several things to me.

Smoking was a form of communication. For Bob and me, smoking was an integral form of communication—something we did together. Post-meal cigarettes were always our favorite, as we would relax, smoke, and talk about our day.

I lived a certain life-style when I smoked. Most of my friends smoked. I'm sure that was not an accident. I chose friends who smoked because I was more comfortable with them. A dear friend of mine was one of those rare people who could pick up a cigarette, smoke it, and then not smoke again for a long time. Smoking didn't dictate a certain life-style for her. However, it did dictate a life-style for me. If I couldn't smoke at someone's home, for example, I'd make an excuse to avoid going there. I usually planned ahead, making certain that I always had extra cigarettes available. I remember a blizzard during which we were snowed in. People couldn't get to work because of the weather. Buses weren't running and planes were grounded. I ran out of cigarettes. I couldn't get my car out of the garage so I hiked to a convenience store just to buy cigarettes.

I used cigarettes as a barrier in interpersonal relationships. At times, when I wanted to make a point, I used cigarettes as a nonverbal communicator. For example, if I wanted to put some distance between myself and another person, I'd light up a cigarette and hold it between us. This served as a sort of "smoke screen," stifling communication, and I could make my point without saying a word. At home, I often used this technique when Bob and I argued.

I used cigarettes to keep a lid on my feelings, especially anger and boredom which are the two feelings that are most difficult for me to contain and control.

Cigarettes became a permission giver for me. If I was tired and needed to take a break, cigarettes gave me permission to sit down, relax, and enjoy a cup of coffee with my cigarette. I couldn't allow myself just to sit down to relax. I needed an excuse, and cigarettes gave me that excuse.

But there were more memories. Some were extremely painful to recall.

Growing aware of smoking's health hazard

During those years of analyzing my smoking habits and occasionally trying to quit, I went through four pregnancies. The first, in 1958, resulted in the birth of a baby girl who died 20 minutes after delivery. During my second pregnancy, I smoked more than ever as I faced a terrifying possibility: what if we lost our second child? I'd heard that cigarette smoking during pregnancy could result in a lower-than-average birth weight, but my fear of my baby dying, ironically, kept me puffing. Sue, born with several health problems, weighed only four pounds, twelve ounces. During the first two years of her life, she had bronchitis so many times that we nearly lost her.

I didn't want to believe that my smoking had affected Sue's birth weight or contributed to her bronchitis. I'd like to believe now that if I had really understood the potentially harmful effects of smoking on my unborn child I would have quit. Sue, constantly exposed to smoking, learned to hate cigarettes. When she was with me as I smoked in the car, she would cough and gag and ask me to throw out my cigarette. I thought she was just being silly and ignored her complaints. Through my negative example, thanks be to God, Sue is now a healthy non-smoker!

I had two miscarriages after Sue's birth. The sad part is I smoked heavily during both pregnancies. In her article, "Women and Children Last?" Jesse L. Steinfeld wrote, "There is a substantial body of evidence which clearly supports the earlier view that maternal smoking during pregnancy harms the unborn child by exerting a retarding influence on fetal growth" (*New York State Journal of Medicine*, Dec. 1983). Sadly, painfully, I have come to believe that my heavy smoking habits most likely contributed to the miscarriages.

I was now convinced that cigarette smoking *could* be a serious threat to health. Just how serious I was soon to find out. My father-in-law, a long-time smoker, developed both emphysema and lung cancer. He had been coughing up blood for a year but hadn't told us. I'll never forget the night the doctor gave us the diagnosis of Dad's biopsy. After hearing the bad news, Bob and I left the room and lit up cigarettes. We didn't know how to handle such terrible news without smoking.

Dad began to have trouble breathing. We watched him struggle for breath as if he was drowning or someone was strangling him. Oxygen was administered through tubes in his nose and respiratory therapy was given. Still he couldn't get enough oxygen. Because eating is difficult when all one's energy is needed just to breathe, Dad became very thin and pale. Finally, he became bedridden, unable to care for himself. In five months' time, we watched a healthy man deteriorate and die. I understood the horrors of emphysema and lung cancer.

Witnessing Dad's death made me intensely aware of what I as a smoker was doing to my body. Dad's death had the same effect on Bob. He began to complain about the tightness in his chest and began decreasing the number of cigarettes he smoked. I began for the first time to *listen* to my body. I started counting how many cigarettes I smoked. I noticed my throat was always sore, and that I couldn't swim underwater as long as I had when I was 21. "Just old age," I told myself. At times I was out of breath, but that, I contended, was due to "too hot" or "too cold" weather. Bob repeatedly told me I had a smoker's cough, but I explained that the cough was left over from last week's cold or that I had something caught in my throat.

The journey continued

The next step came when I finally decided to set a date to quit. "D day" came and I refused to smoke. I was in agony every minute and thought about cigarettes all day. Would I ever think of anything else? When Sue came home from school at three o'clock, she sat at the table to chat with me. How could I carry on a conversation without a cigarette in my hand? I couldn't and I ran for my cigarettes. I quit hundreds of times like that, beginning my day firmly resolved to go without cigarettes, and then lighting up again before the day ended.

I tried another approach, allowing myself two cigarettes a day, one in the morning and one in the evening before I went to bed. This method worked fine for a few days, until I started going to bed at three o'clock in the afternoon just so I could have my second cigarette!

In still another attempt to quit, I gave my cigarettes to a friend who worked in the post office department of a drug store. Each day I stood in line at the postal counter. When my turn came, my friend would give me one cigarette—my allotment for the day. This worked for awhile, until the post office was closed one day and I had to buy a pack of cigarettes.

Finally, I realized that I was looking for some kind of "magic"—an easy way to quit smoking without pain. I admired anyone who could quit. I just didn't know how to do it myself. I knew I needed a special motivation. I

needed something that would give me the will to live—
to choose life instead of cigarettes which would ultimately
destroy me.

One day while reading my Bible, I was struck by a
passage in the book of Isaiah about the folly of worshiping
idols: "From the rest he makes a god, his idol; he bows
down to it and worships. He prays to it and says, 'Save
me; you are my god' " (44:17). I knew at that moment
I had made the cigarette my idol, my god to worship. I
had made the cigarette more important than God, my
family, and my life. I took out a cigarette and studied it.
How could this object, approximately four inches long,
one-quarter-inch in diameter, and composed of white paper wrapped around tobacco, have such control over me?
How could I even take the chance of letting this thing
affect my relationship with God, and ruin my life?

The time finally came when I knew not only that I
should quit smoking but that I *wanted* to quit. I was
participating in a golf tournament. My opponent was
ahead, so I buckled down to try and win the eighth hole—
a long, mean hole. I took it. While walking to number
nine hole, however, I became so out of breath that I had
to let my friend tee off first. I knew then that I had better
take serious action. I visited my doctor and took a breathing test. That was when the word *emphysema* was first
applied to *me*. As I drove home that unforgettable day,
I was terrified. I wanted to throw my cigarettes out the
car window but I didn't have the courage. I needed to
smoke in order to deal with the pain of the diagnosis:
"You're in the early stages of emphysema. . . ." *How
could I possibly live without smoking? How could I live
without the cigarettes which were killing me?* The tears
flowed. I drove home and called my pastor.

If you are a smoker and identified with some of the aspects of my story, then please keep reading. This book can help.

MARILYN VANDER VEEN

Why Do I Smoke?

Whether you are attempting to quit on your own or wish to be a part of a specially designed program such as ours to help you quit, you also will need to ask yourself some questions about *why* you smoke. The following inventory is reprinted with permission from the U.S. Department of Health and Human Services booklet, *Why Do You Smoke?*

WHY DO YOU SMOKE?

Here are some statements made by people to describe what they got out of smoking cigarettes. How often do you feel this way when smoking? Circle one number for each statement. (A = Always. F = Frequently. O = Occasionally. S = Seldom. N = Never.) Important: Answer every question.

		A	F	O	S	N
A.	I smoke cigarettes in order to keep myself from slowing down.	5	4	3	2	(1)

B.   Handling a cigarette is part of the enjoyment of smoking it.   5   4   3   2   (1)

C.   Smoking cigarettes is pleasant and relaxing.   5   4   (3)   2   1

D.   I light up a cigarette when I feel angry about something.   (5)   4   3   2   1

E.   When I have run out of cigarettes I find it almost unbearable until I can get them.   (5)   4   3   2   1

F.   I smoke cigarettes automatically without even being aware of it.   (5)   4   3   2   1

G.   I smoke cigarettes to stimulate me—to perk myself up.   (5)   4   3   2   1

H.   Part of the enjoyment of smoking a cigarette comes from the steps I take to light up.   5   4   3   2   (1)

I.   I find cigarettes pleasurable.   (5)   4   3   2   1

J.   When I feel uncomfortable or upset about something, I light up a cigarette.   (5)   4   3   2   1

K.   I am very much aware of the fact when I am *not* smoking a cigarette.   5   4   (3)   2   1

L.   I light up a cigarette without realizing I still have one burning in the ashtray.   5   4   (3)   2   1

M.   I smoke cigarettes for a "lift."   (5)   4   3   2   1

N.   When I smoke a cigarette, part of the enjoyment is watching the smoke as I exhale it.   5   4   3   2   (1)

O.   I want a cigarette most when I am comfortable and relaxed.   (5)   4   3   2   1

P.   When I feel "blue" or want to take my mind off cares and worries, I smoke cigarettes.   (5)   4   3   2   1

Q. I get a gnawing hunger for a cigarette when I haven't smoked for a while.   (5) 4 3 2 1

R. I've found a cigarette in my mouth and didn't remember putting it there.   (5) 4 3 2 1

How to score

1. Enter the number you have circled for each question in the spaces below, putting the number you have circled for Question A over line A, to Question B over line B, etc.

2. Add the 3 scores on each line to get your totals. For example, the sum of your scores over lines A, G, and M gives you your score on stimulation, lines B, H, and N give you your score on handling, etc.

Totals

$\underline{1} + \underline{5} + \underline{5} =$ _____ 6

A   G   M   Stimulation

$\underline{1} + \underline{1} + \underline{1} =$ _____ 3

B   H   N   Handling

$\underline{3} + \underline{5} + \underline{5} =$ _____ 13

C   I   O   Pleasurable Relaxation

$\underline{5} + \underline{5} + \underline{5} =$ _____ 15

D   J   P   Crutch: Tension Reduction

$\underline{5} + \underline{5} + \underline{5} =$ _____ 15

E   K   Q   Craving: Psychological Addiction

$\underline{5} + \underline{3} + \underline{5} =$ _____ 13

F   L   R   Habit

Scores can vary from 3 to 15. Any score 11 and above is high; any score 7 and below is low.

What kind of smoker are you? What do you get out of smoking? What does it do for you? This test is designed to provide you with a score on each of six factors which describe many people's smoking behavior. Your smoking may be characterized by only one of these factors, or by a combination of factors. In any event, this test will help you identify what you use smoking for and what kind of satisfaction you think you get from smoking.

The six factors measured by this test describe different ways of experiencing or managing certain kinds of feelings. Three of these feeling-states represent the positive feelings people get from smoking: a sense of increased energy or stimulation, the satisfaction of handling or manipulating things, and the enhancing of pleasurable feelings accompanying a state of well-being. The fourth is the decreasing of negative feelings by reducing a state of tension or feelings of anxiety, anger, shame, and the like. The fifth is a complex pattern of increasing and decreasing "craving" for a cigarette, representing a psychological addiction to smoking. The sixth is habit smoking, which takes place in an absence of feeling—purely automatic smoking.

A score of 11 or above on any factor indicates that this factor is an important source of satisfaction for you. The higher your score (15 is the highest), the more important a particular factor is in your smoking and the more useful the discussion of that factor can be in your effort to quit.

A few words of warning: when you give up smoking, you may have to learn to get along without the satisfaction that smoking gives you. Either that, or you will have to find some more acceptable way of getting that satisfaction.

In either case, you need to know just what it is you get out of smoking before you can decide whether to forego the satisfactions it gives you or to find another way to achieve them.

Stimulation. If you score high or fairly high on this factor, it means that you are one of those smokers who is stimulated by cigarettes—you feel that they help wake you up, organize your energies, and keep you going. If you try to give up smoking, you may want a safe substitute: a brisk walk or moderate exercise, for example, whenever you feel the urge to smoke.

Handling. Handling things can be satisfying, but there are many ways to keep your hands busy without lighting up or playing with a cigarette. Why not toy with a pen or pencil? Or try doodling. Or play with a coin, a piece of jewelry, or some other harmless object.

There are plastic cigarettes to play with, or you might even use a real cigarette if you can trust yourself not to light it.

Accentuation of pleasure—pleasurable relaxation. It is not always easy to find out whether you use cigarettes to feel good, that is, to get real pleasure out of smoking (Factor 3) or to keep from feeling so bad (Factor 4). About two-thirds of smokers score high or fairly high on accentuation of pleasure, and about half of those also score as high or higher on reduction of negative feelings.

Those who do get real pleasure out of smoking often find that an honest consideration of the harmful effects of their habit is enough to help them quit. They substitute eating, drinking, social activities, and physical activities—within reasonable bounds—and find they do not seriously miss their cigarettes.

Reduction of negative feelings or "crutch." Many smokers use cigarettes as a kind of crutch in moments of stress or discomfort, and on occasion it may work; the cigarette is sometimes used as a tranquilizer. But the heavy smoker, the person who tries to handle severe personal problems by smoking many times a day, is apt to discover that cigarettes do not help in dealing with problems effectively.

When it comes to quitting, this kind of smoker may find it easy to stop when everything is going well, but may be tempted to start again in a time of crisis. Again, physical exertion, eating, drinking, or social activity—in moderation—may serve as useful substitutes for cigarettes, even in times of tension. The choice of a substitute depends on what will achieve the same effect without having any appreciable risk.

"Craving" or psychological addiction. Quitting smoking is difficult for the person who scores high on the factor of psychological addiction. For that person, the craving for the next cigarette begins to build up the moment they put one out, so tapering off is not likely to work. Such a person must go "cold turkey."

It may be helpful for such a person to smoke more than usual for a day or two, so that the taste for cigarettes is spoiled, and then isolate themselves completely from cigarettes until the craving is gone. Giving up cigarettes may be so difficult and cause so much discomfort that once the person does quit, they will find it easy to resist the temptation to go back to smoking. Otherwise they know that some day they will have to go through the same agony again.

Habit. This kind of smoker is no longer getting much satisfaction from cigarettes. They just light them frequently without even realizing what they are doing. They may find it easy to quit and stay off if they can break built-up habit patterns. Cutting down gradually may be quite effective if there is a change in the way the cigarettes are smoked and the conditions under which they are smoked. The key to success is becoming aware of each cigarette smoked. This can be done by asking yourself, "Do I really want this cigarette?" You may be surprised at how many you do not want.

If you do not score high on any of the six factors, chances are that you do not smoke very much or have not been smoking for very many years. If so, giving up smoking and staying off should be relatively easy.

If you score high on several categories you apparently get several kinds of satisfaction from smoking and will have to find several solutions. Certain combinations of scores may indicate that giving up smoking will be especially difficult. Those who score high on both Factor 4 and Factor 5 (reduction of negative feelings and craving), may have a particularly hard time in going off smoking and staying off. However, there are ways to do it; many smokers represented by this combination have been able to quit.

Others who score high on Factors 1 and 5 may find it useful to change their patterns of smoking and cut down at the same time. They can try to smoke fewer cigarettes, smoke them only half-way down, use low-tar/nicotine cigarettes, and inhale less often and less deeply. After several months of this temporary solution, they may find it easier to stop completely.

You must make two important decisions: (1) whether to try to do without the satisfactions you get from smoking or find an appropriate, less hazardous substitute, and (2) whether to try to cut out cigarettes all at once, or taper off.

Your scores should guide you in making both of these decisions.

Do I Really Want to Quit?

"Benefits" of Smoking

*A*s you have analyzed your smoking habits and your personal reasons for choosing to smoke, you have perhaps been somewhat sidetracked by what you might call "benefits," or "secondary gains," of smoking. Your cigarette may be your friend, your tranquilizer, an "upper," or an aid in communication. Perhaps smoking helps you when you have a decision to make. One salesman who kicked the habit said he noticed that he used the time it took him to remove a cigarette from a pack, tap the filter on his watch face, take his lighter out of his pocket, light up and inhale, as "think time." This ritual was especially helpful, he said, when a customer had a complaint or pushed for a specific delivery date on goods purchased. The salesman's *preparation for smoking* provided a cushion time during which he could think and formulate a good answer. For this particular salesman this cushion was an attractive benefit of smoking.

Other secondary gains derived from smoking might include control of weight, the pleasing taste and aroma of cigarettes, or the feeling of sexiness or attractiveness the smoker may feel comes with smoking.

FACING THE ISSUES

Perhaps you have trouble giving up smoking because it has become part of your routine, or of what is *familiar* to you. Pete is a good example of how hard it is to change what is familiar. Every morning, precisely at the same time, Pete began his ritual: walk out of the house, open the garage door, get into the car, put the key in the ignition, light a cigarette, start the car. After Pete quit smoking he became confused as to how to start his car. The first morning after quitting he found he couldn't start the car because something was missing. Then, he remembered that he didn't smoke. He had to rethink the process of how to start the car. Another example is Genny, who always had a cigarette the minute she jumped out of bed. When she didn't smoke she found she had spare time. Her solution to that problem was to sleep a little later. Smoking is a part of your routine of life, and to change routine takes patience and time.

Perhaps change is difficult because there is a *fear of the problems brought on by success*. If you succeed at quitting you will also have to control your own weight, handle your own stress, and on and on. You will have nothing to lean on or to blame if things go wrong. Thus, you will have to assume more *responsibility* for your actions, and that takes work and commitment.

Guilt is still another reason why change is so difficult. Some people set unrealistic standards for themselves; they think they should be perfect. When they fail at these expectations they feel guilty. They feel like failures. Some feel the need for self-punishment, and smoking becomes an unconscious attempt at this. Some feel like helpless victims, unable to help themselves. Because of this attitude, change becomes next to impossible. This, of course, creates more guilt. The smoking issue thus becomes an ongoing cycle.[1]

So we smoke because of the benefits we derive from smoking, because we like what is familiar, because we are afraid of the additional responsibility, or because we don't think ourselves worthy. These negative concepts often get confirmed and become a solid base for who we are. We then believe that change is impossible and continue to smoke. What we have overlooked, however, is that we have given up the wonderful gift God gives us: the gift of life and living it to the fullest.

SMOKING AND SELF-CONFIDENCE

Why do people smoke? What makes them start to smoke? For Marilyn, peer pressure and the fact that she thought smoking was glamorous and sexy were factors. For others, smoking is a response to stress. Rather than looking for creative, healthy ways to deal with stress, they turn to various "outlets," including cigarettes, alcohol, drugs. For some people smoking provides a security—one they feel is necessary in this unstable world where they constantly face social, moral, and political dilemmas. Smoking, they say, "calms my nerves," "helps me think," "enables me to make decisions." For Marilyn, smoking provided self-confidence—a way to feel good about herself and who she was. Security is, of course, of prime importance to most people. We want to feel good about who we are, confident in ourselves, with our peers in the workplace, and in our world. A secure feeling about ourselves and who we are gives us self-confidence and a sense of control—of power—in our lives.

But in our search for self-confidence, we have become slaves, prisoners of nicotine. We have made nicotine an idol which becomes our authority and power. We have lost contact with our ultimate power: God.

What shapes self-confidence? Dr. Wayne Joosse, a professor of psychology at Calvin College, suggests that five major factors contribute to its formation: (1) life experiences (successes and failures); (2) value system (cultural and personal); (3) relationship with parents; (4) relationships with significant others in our life (teachers, peers, neighbors, coaches, counselors, etc.); (5) religious beliefs and experiences.

These five factors also influence the image we have of ourselves. Our success at friendship, business, sports, and love is largely determined by our self-image and how we feel about who we are.[2] For example, if we feel negatively about ourselves, we probably won't be successful in interpersonal relationships, business, or sports. If we feel negatively about ourselves, we probably will feel of little worth. Women sometimes have trouble feeling of worth because our culture insists that for them "slim is beautiful." Thus, if a woman isn't slim she feels as though she doesn't belong. Many will look for ways to become slim, and one possible way is smoking instead of eating. The same thing applies to men. Our culture says that macho men are sports-minded. The cigarette advertising industry picks up on this concept and includes rugged, healthy-looking men in cigarette ads. Thus the man who *isn't* an athlete may not feel very good about himself. Our personal and cultural values influence who we think we should be.

How we feel about ourselves is also influenced by our parents. For example, if we receive a loving message from our parents, then we feel "hugged." If the message is one which says we are a pain in the neck, then we feel rejected. These messages become the foundation for our self-confidence.

Many people start to smoke when they are young. For them, smoking represents a control over their own lives or a symbol of independence. Some smoke because their peers smoke and they want to be part of the group. Others smoke because they feel their life is meaningless and directionless. Dr. David Myers shares in his book, *Psychology*, that many smoke because they have experienced failure and feel depressed.[3]

During the 1940s, movie stars and cigarette ads suggested that people were nobodies unless they smoked—that when smoking they would discover a whole new world, an idea with great appeal at the time. Thus it was that cigarettes became associated with pleasure. Phrases such as "cocktail and cigarette" or "coffee and cigarette" were seen as a package—a package used for having a good time. Many people, searching for pleasure, picked up the package; thus nicotine, alcohol, and caffeine became a part of their everyday life-style and a part of who they were. We became a society of people trying to enhance our self-image.[4] We became a society of people on drugs.

What we discovered, however, was that for the pleasure of smoking we had to pay the price of discomfort when the nicotine wore off. So we smoked again in order to maintain a "high." Some of us increased the amount of cigarettes we smoked to two, three, four, and five packs a day in order to maintain our pleasure. We were never able to achieve the original "high" with repetition of smoking, yet the discomfort—such as the pain of drug withdrawal—remained strong or became stronger. In other words, the more we smoked, the less our pleasure, the more we craved nicotine.[5] After a few years of smoking, most smokers, instead of getting pleasure, end up with a nicotine hangover and a filthy tasting mouth.

Does this sound like you? Did you begin smoking because you experienced failure in past experiences? Because you wanted to be part of the group? Because you wanted your own sense of authority and power? Did you begin smoking because it sounded like fun? Does part of you want to smoke and part of you want to quit?

If you really want to quit smoking, you will have to change, and change begins within. It begins with believing you can do it. David G. Myers in his book, *Social Psychology*, states that people who feel more control over their own lives are "more likely to be nonsmokers (or to successfully stop smoking), to wear seat belts, and to practice birth control (instead of trusting fate). They are more independent and resistant to being manipulated, they are better able to delay instant gratification in order to achieve long-term goals, and they make more money."[6] Those who feel *less* control over their lives usually let *outside* situations control their lives.

Begin now to take smoking out of your life, to take control over your own life by looking within, by trying to understand why you started smoking. Look at your past life experiences, your value system, your relationship with your parents, your relationships with others, and your religious beliefs and experiences and see what part they played in your smoking history. Then ask yourself, Why do I smoke? Do I really want to quit?

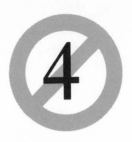

Why Should I Quit?

*J*oan begins each day with a coughing spell and continues to cough throughout the day. Climbing stairs leaves her breathless, as do many other physical activities, and she frequently develops respiratory infections and bronchitis. Joan has the nagging feeling that her pack-a-day smoking habit might contribute to these "minor" irritations. Joan's roommate Angie smokes, too, but she boasts great health and no cough or shortness of breath. She, like Joan, has smoked for several years but she's sure smoking has not affected her health.

Both Joan and Angie *know*, at least on an intellectual level, that smoking is risky business. They've read articles, heard news stories, and even read the Surgeon General's warning on cigarette packages. Joan and Angie *know* the dangers and risks associated with cigarette smoking, including lung cancer and cardiovascular and pulmonary diseases. After much soul searching, both women have decided to quit smoking. They will be amazed at the bodily changes that will take place when they give up cigarettes. Joan will, of course, eventually realize a loss of her smoker's cough, and breathing will be easier. Angie, too, will notice that she feels better in general. Possibly neither will realize what a tremendous gift they have given to themselves by giving up smoking.

As a smoker, you, like Joan and Angie, are most likely aware of the harmful effects of tobacco. You may or may not believe that smoking is affecting you personally. Are you aware of the great benefits that will be yours when you quit smoking? In this chapter, written by John Maurer, M.D., and Dr. John Stewart, we will look at the contents of cigarettes, health risks associated with smoking, the health benefits of quitting, and the stewardship of our bodies.

WHAT'S IN A CIGARETTE?

Just what is in that cigarette that seems to dominate your life? There are literally thousands of different substances in cigarettes, but we focus here on the three major ingredients. The first, nicotine, a primary ingredient in cigarettes, has a definite chemical effect on the body. It increases heart rate and blood pressure, and can cause cardiovascular problems. If you have smoked for any length of time, your body is dependent on nicotine. When you quit smoking you will go through nicotine withdrawal, much as you would for other substances such as alcohol or narcotics. Some people have very little trouble with nicotine withdrawal; others become very ill. Withdrawal symptoms may include nervousness, insomnia, headache, anxiety, tremulousness, and gastrointestinal upset. Symptoms may last from less than a week up to 10 days, depending on how the body reacts to the absence of nicotine.

Roger had smoked for 36 years. When he quit, his withdrawal symptoms were severe. First he developed stomach cramps, then he became constipated. His doctor told him to drink plenty of water and get lots of rest. Roger became light-headed and even confused in his thinking. He claimed that he was outside his body looking in, that the body looked like his but didn't feel like his. Roger was sick for two weeks with his withdrawal.

Smokers who find it nearly impossible to quit smoking because of the intensity of the physical problems may turn to nicotine chewing gum for help. This gum, available only by prescription in this country, contains nicotine and is designed especially for people who have great difficulty giving up tobacco, primarily because of the accompanying nicotine withdrawal symptoms. Such people follow a pattern of quitting, getting sick, then going back to smoking. They may *really* want to quit, but become so ill each time they try that they go back to smoking. The nicotine chewing gum may be used by such smokers to supply the nicotine, upon which their bodies are dependent, while they stop using cigarettes as their source of nicotine. Thus, they can get through the psychological aspects of quitting without experiencing the physical withdrawal symptoms. When they have quit psychologically, while using the gum, they begin gradually to wean themselves off the chewing gum. Although the gum may be helpful to some smokers, it is not helpful to all individuals trying to stop. It doesn't make stopping any easier because it doesn't provide the motivation to quit. The gum does not replace the personal decision that each individual must make in order to quit smoking.

A second major ingredient of cigarette smoke is carbon monoxide, a toxic gas which, in high enough concentrations, is fatal to human beings. Although no one has ever died from cigarette-induced carbon monoxide poisoning, smokers, particularly those who smoke more than two packs a day, have an elevated level of carbon monoxide in their blood. Carbon monoxide impairs the body's ability to carry oxygen from the lungs to the other tissues. The body without enough oxygen, particularly to the brain and heart, is finally unable to survive. Thus, carbon monoxide is harmful to the body because it, like nicotine, is one of the ways smoking increases the risk of cardiovascular problems.

A third major ingredient of cigarettes is tars, which include a whole category of substances. Tars are the major cancer-causing agents in cigarette smoke. They are also responsible for lung damage and may cause emphysema. These substances, when inhaled, are deposited in the lung tissue, impairing the lungs' ability to cleanse themselves and to burn out the tars. The deposited tars will, over a period of years as they are in contact with lung cells, cause these cells to undergo changes that eventually can turn them into cancers or tumors. Experts believe that most cancers, including lung cancers, begin with only one cell or a small group of cells that undergoes change, becomes malignant, and begins to multiply rapidly and erratically.[1]

Cigarette manufacturers, recognizing the growing concern about nicotine and tar in cigarettes, are now producing "low tar" and "low nicotine" cigarettes. These cigarettes are promoted widely with the implication that switching to a low tar and/or low nicotine cigarette will give the smoker a "safe" cigarette. Unfortunately for the smoker, this is not true. First, there is very good evidence that most people who switch to such cigarettes will tend to inhale more and smoke more.[2] Second, there is still enough nicotine, carbon monoxide, tar, and other harmful substances in the cigarette smoke to cause health problems. Manufacturers include additives in order to make low tar/low nicotine cigarettes taste good enough for smokers to use them. Tobacco companies, unlike food and drug manufacturers, are not required by law to divulge what they put into cigarettes. Although some toxic substances in cigarettes have been identified, most others remain unidentified "trade secrets."

There is no "safe" cigarette!

WHAT ARE SMOKING'S HEALTH RISKS?

A five-year study entitled "Closing the Gap" is currently being conducted by the Carter Center of Emory University in Atlanta.[3] According to project co-chairman, William H. Forge, M.D., the purpose of the study is "to close the gap between where we are and where we could be" in regard to national health. The study is focused on what measures we as a nation are taking to improve our overall health. As a part of the study, a list of the most serious health problems in this country was compiled. An analysis of this list led study participants to draw up a second list—a list of "risk factors" which lead to the diseases named on the first list.

Number one on the list of health problems—the primary cause of illness and death in the United States—is cardiovascular disease. Cardiovascular problems are responsible for more than 50 percent of all deaths in the United States, a large number being linked directly with smoking. Number one on the risk factor list is tobacco use. *The leading contributor to death in the United States is tobacco use!* "The Surgeon General's report claims 360,000 deaths a year, or 1,000 a day, are related to tobacco use. . . . It causes more deaths by cardiovascular diseases than by cancer. . . . Nearly a third of all Americans who die of heart disease and stroke are younger than 65, and a quarter of these deaths are attributable to tobacco use."[4]

Think of it—the equivalent of more than two fully loaded 747s per day crashing—without survivors! And our news media hardly notice! Our government subsidizes tobacco growers and our magazines welcome ads. (Imagine that air travel or nuclear power or AIDS began taking an equal number of casualties as does cigarette smoking. What do you suppose would be the public and governmental response?[5]

Smoking promotes hardening of the arteries, the build-up of cholesterol deposits in the arteries. When the deposits occur in the coronary arteries, which are the arteries that supply blood to the heart, an individual can develop angina, or severe chest pains. When an artery becomes completely blocked, a heart attack occurs. Even if the victim lives, the part of the heart muscle that is supplied by that blocked artery dies. Scar tissue forms, limiting the heart's ability to pump blood through the body.

Jim, 57, smoked two packs of cigarettes a day. He suffered from high blood pressure and mild diabetes but never worried much about his health until he began developing chest pains. Tests indicated evidence of heart attack. He received intense medical treatment but his condition deteriorated. He eventually developed heart block and required placement of a pacemaker. Finally his heart no longer was strong enough to pump blood adequately, and he died.

There is *some* good news though. Recent statistics indicate a decrease in the incidence of coronary heart disease and heart attack.[6] That is thought to be due not so much to more efficient coronary care units and new medical developments, but to an increasing recognition of the importance of various risk factors for the development of such health problems—risk factors that include high blood pressure, elevated cholesterol levels, and *cigarette smoking.*

One group that has shown a significant decrease in smoking is males between the ages of 35 and 60.[7] Because males in that age category are far more prone to develop heart disease than are women of the same age, the smoking decrease has spelled a definite decrease in the incidence of coronary heart disease.

The second leading cause of death and illness in this country according to the Atlanta study is cancer. Cancer, especially cancer of the lung, is the disease most often of greatest concern to smokers who have seen pictures of blackened lungs and have heard the lung cancer horror stories.

Ann had been in excellent health all her life. At 64 her major "vice" was cigarette smoking. Despite doctors' suggestions that she quit, she continued her pack-a-day habit. During a routine chest X-ray, doctors detected a nodule on Ann's lung. Tests indicated that the nodule was a primary lung cancer. Surgery was out of the question because of the location of the nodule. Ann has begun radiation therapy, but her chances for a full recovery are very low.

Over 130,000 die each year in the United States from lung cancer.[8] Eighty percent of these deaths are directly linked to tobacco use. Many types of cancer develop without a detectable cause, but there are types, such as lung cancer, that are directly related to cigarette smoking. *This is an avoidable risk!*

Yul Brynner, the famous star of the musical "The King and I," died of lung cancer. Just before he died he said that he wished he could live his life all over again *without smoking;* he attempted to let people know this by filming the last days of his life. His warning was "change your ways or you will end up like me." Other famous people who died prematurely from lung cancer are John Wayne and Steve McQueen. Ironically, Marilyn Vander Veen used movie stars as her model to begin smoking; now movie stars can be used as models to help others give up the destructive habit.

Why is lung cancer becoming more prevalent?

Around the turn of the century, lung cancer was an extremely rare disease, so rare, in fact, that medical textbooks of that time contain scant information about it. What has happened in these last 80 years to cause lung cancer to be the most common cause of cancer death in the United States? Studies very clearly and irrefutably indicate that as cigarette smoking became more widespread, there was a gradual rise in the incidence of lung cancer. This rise reached the point many years ago where lung cancer became the most common cause of cancer death in men. In only the last several years has lung cancer exceeded breast cancer as the most common cause of cancer death in women.[9] An alarming fact is that even 20 years ago lung cancer was number seven on the list of causes of death due to cancer among women in this country, and it was much lower than breast cancer, cancer of the uterus, cancer of the colon, and several others. But in the space of 20 years the incidence has skyrocketed and is continuing to increase among women at an alarming rate. Why? Women in this country did not start smoking in the same numbers as men did until World War II and thereafter. Statistics point out that it takes an average of 20 to 30 years after someone has started smoking for there to be a peak incidence of developing cancer.[10] In other words, if women, as a large group, started to smoke in the 1940s, it wasn't really until the 1970s that this started to show statistically. That was the decade when the dramatic rise occurred—and the rise is continuing.

Other types of cancers of the mouth area, including the larynx (voice box) and the esophagus, and even cancer in organs distant from the mouth and respiratory tract, such as cancers of the bladder, also are increasing in frequency among individuals who smoke.[11] The most significant increase, however, continues to be in the occurrence of lung cancer.

What about chewing tobacco?

The use of chewing tobacco or "snuff" has increased in recent years, perhaps due to the fact that smokers are seeking "safe" tobacco. There is growing evidence, however, linking chewing tobacco with the development of cancer of the mouth or parts of the mouth, such as the tongue, lining cells of the mouth, or larynx.[12] The use of snuff is no safer than the use of cigarettes. Anyone who watches major league baseball knows how popular chewing tobacco is with the ball players. It's a sad commentary on our culture to see that some of the most well-known men—the heroes, in fact, of many young people—are snuff users.

Does smoking have other health risks?

Number seven on the Atlanta study's list as the leading cause of death in the United States is respiratory diseases—still yet another group of diseases directly attributable to tobacco use. Perhaps the best known of these respiratory diseases is emphysema, a destruction of the lung tissues that are responsible for removing carbon dioxide from the body and replacing it with oxygen. The person who develops emphysema is always short of breath and often must use tanked oxygen continuously.

In this dreaded disease the cilia, tiny hairs located in the trachea and main bronchial tubes, are damaged or destroyed by cigarette smoke. These tiny hairs, which help to cleanse the lungs, also serve as infection fighters. Cigarette smoke can damage them to a point where they can be effectively eliminated as functioning cleansers of the lungs. The function of other cleansing cells (macrophages) of the lungs is also inhibited by cigarette smoke. Smoking increases the production of mucus in the lungs, which in turn clogs the lungs and bronchial tubes.

Thus, the smoker *increases* congestion but *decreases* the function of the lungs' cleansing agents. The smoker breathes in tars and other noxious substances, and these in turn destroy the body's main defense mechanism to cleanse itself.

In addition to listing the major causes of illness and death in this country, the Atlanta study looks at what measures we could take to substantially improve our overall health. The far and above number one step recommended for health improvement is: Stop smoking!

WHAT ARE THE HEALTH BENEFITS OF QUITTING?

When you stop smoking, the cilia mentioned above begin to grow back—and fairly quickly. As the cilia grow, they begin to cleanse the lungs. Many people, when they first quit smoking, initially feel worse than they did when they were smoking because they are coughing more. The body is working to expel noxious substances from the lungs. This is a sign that the cilia are again becoming effective cleansing agents.

Even if you have smoked for a number of years and there is some lung damage, once you stop smoking the lungs do begin to repair themselves. If you have developed emphysema to a point where you are on oxygen 24 hours a day, it is, of course, too late for repairs because too much lung damage has occurred.

When you quit smoking your risk of developing cardiovascular diseases, cancer, and respiratory problems begins to drop. Gradually, over a period of years, the risk of a nonsmoker developing cardiovascular disease will rise with age, as it does for all of us as we get older. The risk of a smoker who quits will gradually decrease over the years to a point where it essentially approximates the risk of the nonsmoker.

A recent study points out that, in the case of a heart attack, the risk drop may actually take place over a period of three or four years, dropping a bit each year.[13] The risk drop for lung cancer is approximately 10 years, but even after a single smoke-free year, the risk falls significantly, and after five years the risk is substantially lowered. The important thing is that you stop before irreparable damage has occurred, whether it be cardiovascular problems, cancer, or respiratory problems.

Additional health benefits also occur when you stop smoking. Joan will find herself free, after a time, of her hacking smoker's cough. Climbing stairs will be easier and she will not be so short of breath. Angie, even though she felt she had no problems physically with cigarette smoking, will find that she has much more energy and can do much more than she could previously. Both women will be less susceptible to respiratory infections, coughs, and colds, and will greatly improve their overall health.

STEWARDSHIP OF OUR BODIES

Resolving to quit smoking is a life-affirming decision. We have just explained how smoking is life-threatening. Such a conclusion, medically speaking, is beyond dispute. But underneath the medical reasons, Christians point to even deeper promptings for quitting smoking, namely, the stewardship of our bodies. Let's begin with some biblical beginnings and insights.

The worthiness of physical things is a major theme in the Bible. One recurring melody of the creation narratives in Genesis is the joyous refrain, "God saw all that he had made, and it was very good" (Gen. 1:31). From those awesome beginnings, life is viewed as a good gift from the Creator. We humans did not "create" ourselves, any more than you or I initiated or influenced our own "creation" by our natural parents. Life was breathed into humans from a source beyond ourselves. And all of life was good, very good. Yet along with the *gift of life,* came the *responsibility for life.* Humankind was empowered with God-given capacities to care for the creation, and, as Walter Brueggemann has aptly said, "To see to it that the creation becomes fully the creation willed by God."[14] In short, humans were privileged and empowered by God to become "stewards" over the good creation. Biblically speaking, that stewardship extends to and includes stewardship of our own bodies.

The people in the Old Testament took that responsibility seriously, though not always consistently. They prescribed healthful diets and outlined medicinal procedures (Reread Leviticus in this light!); they affirmed the goodness of human sexuality and set parameters for sexual responsibility and purpose; they even placed the mark of God's covenant (circumcision) in the flesh (Gen. 17:13).

They also believed (and Jesus affirmed) that the Messiah would enable the blind to see, the oppressed to be set free, and the good news to come even to the poor (Isa. 61; see also Luke 4). They sang of the wonder of the human creation, as in Psalm 139: "For you created my inmost being. . . . your works are wonderful, I know that full well. My frame was not hidden from you" (vv. 13-15). Few beliefs of the New Testament people of God are more central than the celebrated words of John, "The Word became flesh and made his dwelling among us" (1:14). Among the most surprising affirmations of the New Testament is the resurrection of the body. A person's body is so delicately precious that the apostle Paul announces that in the new era after Pentecost, our *bodies* become "temples" of the Holy Spirit. "For God's temple is sacred, and you are that temple" (1 Cor. 3:17). The human body is so indispensable to our humanity and the Creator's intention that, in the end times, humans will receive new—and better—bodies with which to worship and serve our Creator-Redeemer Lord (Rev. 21:1-4). In short, from Genesis to Revelation, the human body is understood as a gift from God. As God's people we are given the freedom and responsibility to care for the totality of human life, including our bodies. It is in this large and exalted sense that smoking, an inherently destructive human habit, is contrary to the Creator's intention. It is an addiction to self-destructive behavior, and Jesus reigns that we might have life, not death.

How Can I Change?

*H*ow do ordinary people change? Most of us are creatures of habit. We're addicted to patterns of behavior. As in piano practicing, or driving a stick shift after years of automatic transmission, or pronouncing a new French phrase, or smoking cigarettes, repetition ingrains and routinizes human behaviors. We become willing to change our behavior pattern only when some significant, conscious dissonance emerges and disturbs us. A persistent annoyance—"Your smoking stinks up this room!"—or an impending crisis—"The doctor says I have emphysema, and I gotta quit!"—is usually a prerequisite for abandoning those patterns. Change, therefore, always carries a challenge. It always demands courage because some pain will accompany altering established patterns. New ways, they say, make new muscles sore.

When one dares to change from a smoker to a non-smoker, a tough challenge, but not an impossible one, confronts us. Many of us have established smoking pat-terns—rituals—for years. These behavior patterns are wedded to certain chemical addictions that make quitting even harder and more painful. Personal behaviors, chem-ical involvement, and social "pressures" make for a pow-erful set of obstacles to overcome. But kicking the nicotine habit can be, and is being, accomplished by ordinary people in some ordinary ways.

FIVE PRINCIPLES OF CHANGE

Listed below are five principles, suggested by John Stew-art, that may guide you as you begin your change.

Alter your regular behavior patterns

How you "feel" about giving up cigarettes will most likely *not* lead you to quit. You may have accepted the fact that you *want* to quit, *should* quit, or *must* quit because of health problems, but this knowledge and the feelings associated with it will not make you a nonsmoker. Your attitudes about smoking will not be challenged until you intentionally *alter the patterns and rituals* that support and endorse your smoking habit.

Once you have decided to quit smoking, you must begin to take action to *alter your behavior habits and patterns*. For example, take a new route to work, go for a walk after meals (instead of settling down in your favorite easy chair with a cigarette or pipe), pursue a new hobby, and so on. Begin by changing your "public" world. When little changes begin to occur in your public world, then little changes will begin to take place in your private world. Like salespeople with a new product, the more they "talk up" the product, the more convinced they become of its worth. It is akin to the phrase, practicing what we preach. Your attitudes and motives about smoking will rarely be challenged until you intentionally alter the patterns that support your smoking habit. Actions condition attitudes.

Perhaps you will choose a more drastic way of quitting—going "cold turkey," perhaps on a weekend retreat. Whichever route you take, you will see that actions do condition attitudes. You can "snap the trap" by *altering the regular behavior patterns* that surround your smoking habit. Doing empowers motivation to continue doing.

Reward small accomplishments

Reward your successes! Even the slightest change of a pattern of behavior that leads to *not* smoking should be rewarded promptly and imaginatively. Candy may not be dandy for you, but you must find ways to give yourself a treat when you succeed. Be creative! A fly-fisherman added one new dry fly to his collection for each day he didn't smoke. A woman treated herself with a trip to the hairdresser for each week she went without smoking, justifying the expense by comparing it to the cost of her two-pack-a-day smoking habit. Treat yourself when you succeed even a little. Rewards motivate! Quitting the smoking habit is tough, and you deserve a reward for each step you take toward becoming a nonsmoker.

Set small, attainable goals

There is a ton of wisdom in the proverb, "inch by inch, life's a cinch!" You do not have to quit smoking in one big "gulp." Set small, definite, attainable, yet realistic goals. Instead of saying, "I'm giving up smoking right now and forever," say, "today I will not smoke before noon." If even a half day without cigarettes seems impossible, perhaps one hour, or even ten minutes, is a better goal. Whatever the goal, when you have arrived at it—smokeless—reward your accomplishment and immediately set another goal. If you attained your goal of getting through the morning without smoking, perhaps your next goal will be, "I will not smoke before supper."

Altering your smoking patterns for short, attainable periods of time empowers you and reinforces your resolve to keep trying—to keep inching your way toward becoming a nonsmoker. You may not win the war immediately but you are winning battles! When you are able to go smokeless for one whole day, stretch a bit and resolve not to smoke for two days or more. Be sure that your goal is definite but small enough to be within *your* reach.

If you fail, forgive yourself. You are not perfect. Regroup by setting a new goal, perhaps a smaller, more attainable one. And when you reach that goal, reward yourself. You deserve it!

Join a group

If you are not aware of a group of people that is trying to quit smoking, form one. Smoking has social dimensions. Peers most likely helped you to start smoking and peers now can help you to quit. Others can help to accomplish what might be too demanding to do alone. Countless other "change-agent" programs, perhaps none more savvy than Alcoholics Anonymous, know the wisdom of group therapy. Joining a group to help you kick the habit is not an admission of weakness, but an acknowledgment that you are a social creature.

Regular participation with others in a group geared to stop smoking provides three critical ingredients that are unattainable to you alone. First, such groups provide a sense of empathy. Your new friends *know* your struggles firsthand. Trust, acceptance, and camaraderie flow from your common weakness, not from your strengths. Second, the group provides approval of your attainments. Others can help reinforce your resolve to attain your goals. Since smoking is such a "social" event, the group's encouragement will serve as a powerful reward. And you'll strengthen your own determination by encouraging others. New behaviors breed new attitudes. Third, the group is a place of accountability. Success usually comes more easily when we are accountable to others, especially in an environment of acceptance and encouragement. Participation in regularly scheduled group meetings firms up private resolutions.

Ask God regularly to help you quit smoking

The stop-smoking approach advocated in this book grew out of experiences of people in a Christian community. Those who have, over the years, participated in our program and have contributed to this book believe that God's power is a transcendent, loving power that promotes life. Smoking promotes death. We believe that the power unleashed in the resurrection of our Lord Jesus is available for all persons. "I have come that they may have life, and have it to the full" (John 10:10).

Smoking is not so much immoral as it is tragic and, well, dumb. We love life and living, yet smoking promotes the ending of life. As you begin the change process, ask God to intervene and to help you change. Pray often and regularly. We who have been successful in our efforts to quit smoking know the power of prayer. Some of us have had dramatic results. Several have experienced a revolutionary withdrawal of need and desire to smoke. Others have struggled in a more gradual way: succeeding, back-sliding, trying again. There is no *one* model or way, but we attest that God is in our midst bringing life. More often than not, most of us experience the power of God through other concerned Christian persons. Their stead-fastness and love are the channels for God's life-giving changes. As the apostle Paul put it, "I can do everything through him [Christ] who gives me strength" (Phil. 4:13).

The availability of God's help will probably require one more strategy on your part. Few of us experience God directly and in isolation. Rather, most experience the presence and power of God when God is "incarnated" to us through other persons. To participate in the Christian community, the body of Christ, means to engage in friendship with other Christians. Friends not only care about us, they care enough to keep us honest and ac-countable. Resolving to stop smoking, like altering any other ingrained habit, will require "tough-love" encoun-ters with a trusted friend.

A time-tested strategy is to ask a friend to enter a partnership with you; to keep you accountable to your resolution; to "hear your confession" of failures; to affirm your hard-won successes; and, best of all, to pray regularly for your kicking the smoking habit. Such a soul-friend will rejoice with you when you succeed, and suffer with you when you fail. That is how the Bible envisions the Christian community to be linked and energized. (See 1 Corinthians 12:14-26.) The common wisdom of Christian people is straightforward: don't try to go it alone. Allow God to engage you *through* other persons—especially a good friend. That is what one child meant when she said that "a friend is God with a face."

These five principles for change—alter your regular behavior patterns, reward small accomplishments, set small, attainable goals, join a group, and ask God regularly to help you quit smoking—are meant to be holistic, that is, involving the entire person: body, mind, and spirit. Smoking affects *all* dimensions of us. Our experience has proven that when you "wage the battle" holistically you'll be more likely to win. Power to you!

Make three copies of the five principles, and place one copy on your refrigerator at home, one copy somewhere in your workplace, and one copy on your bathroom mirror. These copies will be a reminder of ways to cope while giving up smoking.

John Stewart relates a personal experience to round out these principles on how to change.

Knowing how to change and wanting to change are not on the same level. Knowledge doesn't always provide sufficient (or efficient) motivation. But change is often prompted after a deep personal encounter. That is what happened to me. I had been a pipe smoker for years. Holes in my trousers and constant throat clearing demonstrated my habit to all. One morning, while trying to find a pen in my junior high school son's book bag, I discovered a pack of cigarettes. A curious rage crested within me. When he came downstairs I pounced on him saying, "Where did these cigarettes come from? How long have you been smoking? Don't you know how dumb it is to smoke?"

He just stared, mostly in disbelief. Then he unleashed his zinger on me. "Why should you get on my case?" he said. "You smoke!" Instantly I knew for his sake and mine that I had to change. So I gathered my wits and fatherly composure and said, "Let's make a bargain. If you quit, I will too. If you will help me, I'll help you and I promise if I start up again, I'll tell you. Will you promise the same?" He said he would. We shook on it and left resolved to change. And we did.

Your "Smoker-Within"

*A*s you begin to take steps toward becoming a non-smoker, it is important that you put aside all pre-conceived notions of what quitting is like. Start fresh! Try to forget the stories you've heard about the difficulties involved with quitting. Concentrate on *now* and prepare your mind to develop a whole new base of information about cigarette smoking and a stronger foundation of facts on which to begin your recovery from cigarette addiction. Susie Heritage shares some ideas about confronting the "smoker-within," the part of you that wants you to keep smoking.

PERSONAL RESPONSIBILITY

To stop smoking is an issue of *personal responsibility*. You are not a helpless victim. No person or situation can *make* you smoke. The only reason you will smoke is because you *choose* to smoke. Likewise, there is no magic to help you stop smoking. How easy and simple it would all be if this were so, but it's not. It's crucial to understand that.

Just as it is your responsibility to smoke or not to smoke, it is your responsibility to be honest with yourself about the number of cigarettes you smoke and the cost to your health. Smokers tend to fool themselves, perhaps in an effort to lessen their problem, but it is important to be honest with yourself on this subject.

Smokers sometimes tend to project their problems onto other people. For example, "that person" or "that situation" made me smoke. When Barb was trying to quit smoking, she would often wake in the morning with great resolve that today was the day to quit. She would do well for a while but as the day wore on and not smoking became more difficult, she would unconsciously begin to look for an excuse to smoke. Often that excuse would be something she and her husband disagreed about, and she would trot off to the convenience store for her cigarettes saying to herself, "How can I quit when *he's* going to act like that!" In reality, of course, she was *choosing* to smoke and blaming her bad decision on her husband.

No one and nothing can make you smoke. You only will smoke if you choose to smoke. The wonderful part is you have a *choice!* Just as you may choose to smoke, you may choose *not* to smoke. With every cigarette you pick up, you have a conscious choice to make. Awareness of "choice" is important because smokers tend to think of themselves as "helpless" when it comes to cigarettes. You must come to realize that you are not helpless, but that you have a choice, and that you can choose *not* to smoke.

Ownership

Part of owning up to how much you smoke and the threat to your health is owning up to the smoker that lives within you. In a sense, once you are a smoker, you will always be a smoker. You know how the cigarette tastes, how it feels, how it smells, how to hold it, how to inhale, and so on. When you stop smoking, you will not instantly forget all these things. They will be a part of you even though you may never smoke again. That part of you (the smoker that lives within) will always know how to smoke. Awareness of this fact is important because that smoker-within can sabotage your efforts to quit and you may find yourself with a cigarette between your lips and wondering how it got there. A part of you wants badly to smoke, even if you might die because of smoking.

Another important part of owning the smoker-within is verbalization. When you want a cigarette, talk about it. Share your feelings with others, write them in a journal, or just say them aloud to yourself. Don't withdraw and repress the desire to smoke. Express the desire and get it outside yourself. The better you understand the smoker part of you, the more equipped you will be to stop smoking. Part of what you must own up to are the hard truths about the characteristics of the smoker-within. You might even have to ask yourself why you want to die, since that may be part of the truth about your destructive behavior. The important thing is if you refuse to do something, admit it. In other words, your "I *can't* quit smoking" is really "I *won't* quit smoking!" Own the problem and realize that the choice is yours.

Motivation and awareness

You must also understand that to stop smoking is a matter of *motivation and awareness*. We are not talking about "grin-and-bear-it" willpower. Self-education and insight are more important in the stop-smoking process than is willpower. Perhaps the strongest, most powerful motivator to stop smoking is self-preservation.

As a smoker, there are two parts of you. One part wants to smoke. Right now that part of you, the smoker-within, might feel very strong, very large. The other part of you, the part that wants to stop smoking, might feel weak and small. In your process to quit smoking, the nonsmoker within will begin to grow. When it eventually becomes stronger than the smoker part, *you will quit!* That's why it is a matter of motivation and education, and not just willpower. The conflict between these two parts of you is the motivational issue.

THE PROCESS AND THE PARADOXICAL THEORY OF CHANGE

Just how does this process of moving from smoker to nonsmoker work, you may wonder. Change will come as you continue to learn more about the smoker part of you. As you better understand the smoker, the stronger the nonsmoker will become. The transfer of power from smoker to nonsmoker will come when, in your quitting process, the nonsmoker finally becomes stronger than the smoker. This theory is based on the paradoxical theory of change that says you only move toward Point B (nonsmoker) by becoming totally aware of who and what you are at Point A (smoker). In other words, you can push and shove yourself all day toward Point B and never move. But when you immerse yourself into really understanding yourself at Point A (smoker), movement toward Point B (nonsmoker) becomes much easier. You must know what you're doing right now and how you're doing it if you hope to change. That's why it's important to say, "Right now, I want to smoke," and then ask yourself, "Why?"

Share it, write about it, express it! Ask: "What's happening? Why do I want to smoke now? What do I need
to learn about my smoking? What do I believe this cigarette will do for me? How else might I be able to do that
for myself?" If you try to repress the "urge" to smoke,
without expressing your feelings, you may sabotage your
good intentions by reasoning, "Well, maybe just one
won't hurt." Part of the truth you might need to learn
is that for you maybe one *will* hurt because that one will
lead to two, three, and, perhaps, an entire pack. In any
case, the more you understand yourself as a smoker, the
more you can help yourself become a nonsmoker.

As you move toward becoming a nonsmoker, remember
that to quit smoking is indeed a *process*, not an event.
Cheryl's process is an example of this. Cheryl had just
passed the bar and was working as an apprentice lawyer
for one of the local judges when she decided that that
was the time to quit smoking. She was instructed the first
day of the clinic (Monday) to get rid of her cigarettes,
hide the ashtrays, and give or throw away lighters and
other paraphernalia. So on Tuesday, she threw all her
cigarettes in the trash can, went to work, and at night
reported to the group at the clinic of her success. Everyone
cheered and praised her good deed. However, when
Cheryl returned home she went directly to the trash can
and retrieved the cigarettes. She smoked them one by
one until they were all gone. She then took off her coat
and settled down to the tasks at hand. She hasn't smoked
since and has been instrumental in helping many others
quit smoking. She couldn't quit smoking until she had
smoked that last cigarette. That was part of her process.

Most likely, you did not smoke your first cigarette and
just instantly love it and inhale it. You probably had to
work at learning how to hold the cigarette, how to flick

the ashes, how not to turn green, how to inhale, and so on. Just as you worked at learning *how* to smoke, you must work at learning how *not* to smoke. For a part of your life you have lived the life-style of a smoker. Now you will be restyling your life to that of a nonsmoker. You will learn how to do very familiar things all over again in a new way, as a nonsmoker. You will learn how to talk on the phone as a nonsmoker, how to carry on a conversation, or how to drink a cup of coffee without a cigarette in hand. Quitting thus becomes an educational process, a growing process during which you will discover interesting, new facts about yourself. You most likely will learn that you are a much stronger person than you believe you are right now.

You must understand that the process of quitting is a very individual, very personal one. No two people quit in exactly the same way. You can't compare the specifics of your process to the specifics of anyone else's, although there may certainly be similarities to share. Above all, you should not expect that because something was true for someone else, it will be true for you.

Keep trying! As you work through the process, find someone to work with you, either individually or through the group support that a stop-smoking program such as the one suggested in this book can provide.

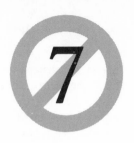

Building
Self-confidence

*A*s you work through your process of quitting smoking, the question of "Who am I?" will arise. As you confront your smoker-within, as you try to restyle your life to that of a nonsmoker, the image you had of yourself will change. This is a growing, but painful, process. The questions you need to ask yourself are: "Can I change my self-esteem?" "Can I overcome negative feelings?" Praise God, the answer is yes!

Smoking and self-confidence were dealt with in some measure earlier in this book (see pp. 32-35). Although it is very difficult to build self-confidence, it can be done. What it will take is a strong commitment. It will take more than simply reading a book or listening to a lecture; it will take total commitment, goals, plenty of hard work, and an abundance of prayer. Marilyn Vander Veen shares some ideas about building self-confidence.

First, believe that you have the ability to quit smoking. Second, try not to get discouraged when everything isn't as you planned. Be flexible. Try different avenues of quitting. Use your imagination. Third, look within for inner strengths. Ask the Lord for strength and guidance. Then apply the five principles and confront your smoker-within as suggested in Chapters 5 and 6. Look for ways to build a new and strong self-confidence, without smoking. Day by day, as you give up smoking, you will feel a sense of pride and self-worth in your accomplishments.

Beth, a shy, prim, and proper retired English professor disliked herself as a smoker. She viewed smoking as slow-motion suicide. When her doctor advised her to quit smoking, Beth wasn't sure she could. She had smoked for many years and she wasn't certain that an "old dog" could learn new tricks. She loved life and was willing to try, so she signed up for our weekend retreat. Rather than the horrid experience she had anticipated, Beth underwent an awakening. She slowly began to take responsibility for her smoking habit. She began to rediscover some of her special gifts, one of which was her wonderful sense of humor. She learned to laugh herself through some difficult times and even began teaching the other participants how to laugh at themselves. Beth changed her self-image: she became outgoing, a little eccentric, and in charge of her smoking habit. Interestingly, Beth also took up fishing during her free time at the retreat. This sport, new to Beth, opened up a whole world for her. Beth, even as a retired professor, was developing a new self-image.

How does one become a whole new person?

1. Begin by looking again at why you smoke. Make your own personal list of why you smoke. This will get you in touch with your smoker-within.

2. Make a list of how you see yourself or your self-image. Make sure to list your strengths and weaknesses.

3. Take the Myers-Briggs Type Indicator test (see p. 145), a tool to help you understand what your basic personality makeup is. This test, based on Carl Jung's theory of types of human personalities, reveals psychological preferences, such as thinking or feeling as you relate to the world, and extrovert (outgoing and people-oriented) or introvert (needing your own personal space to think things through). In childhood, we learned to develop preferences, and as adults, some of them become clearcut. This test is used by the stop-smoking program to help participants understand a little more about themselves.

4. Look for ways to strengthen your self-confidence. The following are four techniques or rules suggested by Alan Loy McGinnis in his book, *Confidence: How to Succeed at Being Yourself*,[1] which can help you grow and develop stronger self-confidence while giving up smoking.

FOUR TECHNIQUES FOR SELF-CONFIDENCE

Focus on Your Potential Instead of Your Limitations

Amy, a junior in high school, had a slight physical defect. Her friends were all athletes. Amy could not keep up with her friends in sports and felt inferior because of it. However, a wise teacher pointed out Amy's strong points: her ability to play musical instruments and her love of music. Amy stopped comparing herself to her friends and grew in her own talent. She not only became a strong person within but was able to enjoy and support her friends as well. Because of her own inner strength, Amy never started smoking. She had developed strong self-confidence and didn't need nicotine or alcohol.

We often get so hung up on our defects that we forget to look at the whole picture of ourselves. We all have weaknesses. "The trick," says McGinnis, "is to determine which ones are improvable, then get to work on those and forget about the rest."[2] Remember that people with high self-confidence may have more weaknesses than those with low self-confidence; they just don't dwell on them. Spend your energy on ways to grow and achieve as a new person.

Find something you like to do and do well, then do it over and over

McGinnis feels that a strong self-image will develop when you identify your talent. The next step is to practice and improve this talent until you are very good at it. This will help you identify a place in the world—a place where you feel you belong.

Take a look at your strengths and ask yourself where you want to spend your energy. What talent do you want to work at? If people really like to do something, they will spend hours at it, happily. Remember, however, that although you may make mistakes and fall on your face, this is how you learn.

You may even need to take on a new identity. We all are made up of many people, many roles. For example, most of us are or have been parent, spouse, counselor, worker, friend, student, volunteer, and so on. If you have used your energy in one area of your identity and it didn't feel comfortable, then try on another part of your identity. For example, Mary, a full-time homemaker who used all of her energy to maintain her home and family, reflected little enthusiasm for being a homemaker, and her self-image was poor. When Mary quit smoking, she decided to go back to college to "try on her new identity." Her confidence soared as she uncovered a new talent: physical therapy. She is now working with young people with disabilities and is extremely happy because she is using her energy in a way that makes her feel good about herself. Interestingly, Mary's family has picked up on her enthusiasm, and is seeking ways to discover their own talents. Mary has become their model.

Dick, a successful surgeon, is another example of changed identity. While going through the process of quitting smoking and trying to understand better who he was, Dick, decided to change his career. He had always dreamed of teaching—that is, teaching young men and women the art of making a sick person healthy by surgery. He knew he wouldn't make the money that he had made as a surgeon but he would have the satisfaction of knowing he could pass his gifts on to young medical students. Dick became a very good teacher and a much-in-demand, renowned lecturer. He found new gifts.

Some people take a long time to discover their talents. For many, it takes a lifetime. So keep working at trying to discover yours and don't be afraid to try some new ideas. When you find the right niche—the thing you enjoy doing—then do it over and over again until you are really good. You will soon have increased your feelings of personal worth.

Replace fear of failure with clear pictures of yourself functioning successfully and happily

Julia, a hard-core smoker, knew she was developing a health problem due to her smoking. She was out of breath when climbing stairs, swimming, or walking briskly. She knew she *should* quit smoking but she wasn't sure she *could* or really *wanted* to give up her habit. Julia had been a smoker for many years; she couldn't even imagine herself as a nonsmoker. Julia finally came to our clinic for help. The instructor asked the participants to relax and then walk themselves mentally through a normal day of their life, rehearsing all of their activities as they did them, cigarette in hand. When they had finished, she asked them to repeat the process, but *without* cigarettes in the picture. It was during the last part of the exercise that Julia could see herself not smoking. She lost her fear of trying to quit and eventually became a successful nonsmoker.

Julia actually worked through a process called "visualization" when she pictured herself living without cigarettes. Visualization is explained in Chapter 10, "How to Handle Stress—without Smoking!" Imagine walking through a day of your life—first smoking, then not smoking. This exercise will help you have a clear picture of yourself as a nonsmoker.

Sometimes in order to go forward, we must first go backward. Visualization can help you understand some of your past as well as help you look at your future. In looking at your past, remember that your self-image was formed at an early age. It was formed by parents, teachers, relatives, peers, ministers, and so on. Who you are today was formed by the messages you received by these people. If you feel unhappy about yourself you might have to ask the question, "Do I have a distorted view of my past experiences?" Evaluate your past, form a more accurate reconstruction of it, and then look at it more objectively. In other words, heal some old wounds. The past might have been damaging to you, but are you going to feel sorry for yourself for the rest of your life? Are you going to spend the rest of your life trying to get approval from others, or trying to get even, or are you going to come to terms with the past and move on to the area where God wants you to be?[3]

Visualize yourself as a healthy human being. Visualize those tiny hairs called cilia beginning to grow back and healthy lungs beginning to emerge. Visualize yourself as a successful, talented, in-control nonsmoker. Visualize yourself full of energy, taking the message of your success, with God's help, to the world! Then thank God that you had the choice.

Cultivate people who help you grow

Bill, who quit smoking through a program at his office, used his stop-smoking support group as a sounding board and a tool to help him grow and change. One day, shortly after Bill had quit smoking, he found that someone had parked in his assigned parking space at the office, thereby forcing Bill to park quite some distance away. He was so angry that his spot had been taken and that he had had to walk so far that he decided to have a cigarette. He stole a cigarette from a friend, checked to see if he was followed, and went out in the farthest corner of the factory behind some stacked barrels to smoke the cigarette. He stuck it in his mouth and reached in his pants for a light. He had forgotten a match! Bill laughed at himself and threw the cigarette away, but he learned something about himself that day. He learned that he handled anger with a cigarette. Sharing the experience with his stop-smoking support group helped Bill to verbalize the problem. Bill was building a network of supportive relationships.

One of the first questions we ask people after they have completed a stop-smoking clinic or retreat is if they have a support system. This support can be a spouse, children, friends, minister, or the support group formed after a stop-smoking program. Many smokers consider their cigarette to be a friend—a very good friend. A grief process follows the loss of the cigarette, and it helps to have someone with whom to share this grief.

As you focus on stronger self-confidence, realizing your gifts and envisioning your successes, it will be so much more meaningful if you have someone with whom to share your successes. Look around at your community—at the people who share your life—and find those who will help you grow and become a nonsmoker.

Most importantly, look at your relationship with God. Are you honoring the privilege of being created in God's image? As you map out your future, are you including God in your plans, thinking about where you fit into God's plan? One of the most wonderful forms of support is prayer. When you give God your problems, ask for strength, and feel the love God has for you, a wonderful peace will come upon you. God is your perfect support.

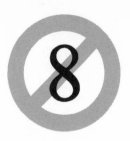

Goal Setting and Keeping a Journal

Y ou've come a long way, baby!" This phrase, most often identified with a particular cigarette advertising campaign, can now begin to apply to *you* in a new and exciting way. You *have* come a long way, for you have finally begun the quit-smoking process. You have begun the journey! No one makes a journey without preparation. If you were planning a cross-country automobile trip from New York to Los Angeles, you would plan your route, gather maps to help keep you on course, and perhaps set daily mileage goals. In short, you would know not only *where* you were going, but precisely *how* you would get there. Simply getting in your car and heading west would not be sufficient. You would most likely wander off course, take wrong turns, and experience a very long, tedious trip.

Just as in traveling you need a plan, so in the quitting-smoking process you need a plan. We recommend two very significant tools as you begin. The first is *goal setting*. The second, *keeping a journal*. Both of these tools will serve as tremendous aids as you work through the quitting process.

SAYING GOOD-BYE

You wouldn't leave on a trip without saying good-bye to family and friends. So also you will find it most helpful to say good-bye to your cigarettes, pipe, or cigars before you begin the quitting process. A very helpful way to say good-bye is through a letter. Gil VandenBerg, who attended a stop-smoking clinic, wrote such a letter:

Dear Phony Friend,

When I was a young man, I found you in the gutter. You were kind of ugly, but most of my friends thought that I was quite somebody because I picked you up, so I let you come home with me. That was a mistake. I knew I had to get rid of you sometime, but it didn't bother me then. However, now is the time you must leave.

I hate to do it because over all these years, I have really come to like you a lot. When we first met, you were like a puppy dog that was fun to play with. As we grew older you would follow me wherever I played. You became such a close friend that I even took you with me when I went to high school. Since I graduated, you have been my constant companion.

Without realizing it, you have become like a seeing eye dog to me. I haven't been able to go anywhere without you. I haven't been able to have a meal or a drink without you being there. You are there the first thing in the morning and the last thing every night. I have become so dependent on you that it makes me mad.

But now, my phony friend, the truth has come out—you truly are a phony. I don't need you at all. In fact, I will be much better off without you. Even though I'm very angry with you, I still like you. You will be missed I'm sure. But you must go, *now!* After all, you are not my seeing eye dog, you are just a dirty ole cigarette.

Gil

GOAL SETTING

As you work toward giving up cigarettes you are doing more than just working at becoming a nonsmoker. You are actually beginning a new life-style in which you will no longer need a cigarette to guide you through every activity you are involved in. As a smoker, you have a smoker's life-style—a life-style which is controlled by your smoking habit. For example, you choose other smokers as friends, your activities include smoking, and cigarettes are within your grasp at all times. When you quit smoking, your life-style will change. Normal routines will become disrupted, anxieties will mount, tempers flare, and feelings of dismay will overwhelm you. Fight back! Consider ways in which you might counter your anxieties, temper, or depression.

Just as you do not go on a trip without a plan, you cannot begin a new life-style without a plan—without goals. As mentioned earlier (pp. 51-52), *set goals*. We recommend setting goals in three areas: exercise, play, and purpose of life, goals that will help you begin a new life-style.

Exercise goals

The function of exercise goals is to direct energies outward, alleviating the buildup of stress that will most likely occur as you begin to think about giving up cigarettes.

When selecting an exercise goal that is just right for you, consider the time you have available in your schedule for exercise. *Daily* exercise is best. Also, consider your state of fitness. Don't expect to be able to run five miles the day you begin your plan. Consult your doctor about an exercise goal that is suitable for you. Be sure to choose a form of exercise that you will enjoy—one that you will look forward to with joyful, eager anticipation.

Sam hated exercising but knew how important it was to relieve built-up stress and anxieties while giving up smoking. So he organized a group of people in his office into a lunch hour walking group. For the first week, 20 people walked approximately one mile, taking various routes. By the end of the month, the group was walking three miles each day. Exercise became an enjoyable daily activity for Sam.

Play goals

Choose activities for play that will be pure fun. When seeking such activities ask: What are my hobbies? How do I relax? What is really fun for me? How much free time do I have? Whether you choose to read, listen to music, or take a walk in the woods, be sure your play goals reflect pure leisure. Relax.

Sarah found she had gained a tremendous amount of time when not smoking. Instead of giving in to boredom, she decided to start afternoon sessions of jazz, something she loved doing. She played a guitar, one neighbor played the drums, another the sax. They practiced daily and became good—so good that they were asked to play for various parties. These jazz sessions reflected pure leisure for Sarah.

"Purpose of life" goals

These goals represent direction in your life. You might consider going back to college, spending more time with your family, changing jobs, making new friends, or scheduling additional time for prayer and meditation. Before setting a goal in this area, spend some time analyzing your present life-style, evaluating the way it is now, and what you might like to change or improve upon.

Kevin had his support group rolling on the floor with laughter while sharing his purpose of life goals with them. Kevin, a ski resort manager, decided he needed to spend more time with his family. He decided to do this by helping his wife around the house. He asked his wife for odd jobs. She suggested he wash the dishes . . . but he broke nearly every dish in the house! His wife shooed him out of the kitchen. Kevin then decided to assist with the laundry. He scooped up a pile of dirty clothes and put them in the washer. The only trouble was he threw red, green, black, blue, and whites all together. He is now wearing greenish, bluish, pink T-shirts. When his wife asked him to go back to smoking, Kevin decided to change his purpose of life goals.

Record your goals in a notebook, perhaps in a chart form such as in the following illustration. Set goals for three months, the next six months, the next nine months, the next year. Your goals should be such that they move you in the direction of wholeness and wellness.

	Play	Exercise	Purpose of Life
3 months	_____	_____	_____
6 months	_____	_____	_____
9 months	_____	_____	_____
12 months	_____	_____	_____

REWARDING YOURSELF: A TOKEN PLAN

Although saying good-bye, setting goals, and beginning a new life-style may be enough to move some people down the road to freedom from cigarettes, other people will do better with a reward system. Small rewards along the way might be just the motivation you need to keep you working toward your goals (see pp. 51-52). You might set up a "token plan,"[1] by which you reward yourself daily with reinforcers (slips of paper, tokens). Later, these may be exchanged for a reward, such as a new dress or suit, a tennis racket, or a trip to Florida.

Behavior Desired/Tokens Received

Walk 4 blocks	1 token
Walk 2 miles	3 tokens
Exercise class (15 minutes)	2 tokens
Tennis (1 hour of doubles)	4 tokens
Swim (4 times around the pool)	2 tokens

Redemption Value of Tokens

Dinner at a restaurant	50 tokens
A movie	20 tokens
A new dress	70 tokens
A new golf club	100 tokens

You may reward yourself for every goal met. Collecting will be fun! Try setting up your own token program. You'll see that it makes exercise, play, and purpose of life goals more fun to work toward.

KEEPING A JOURNAL

Some travelers like to keep journals while on the road, although they don't usually call these records journals.

Perhaps they think of them as mileage logs, or lists of the different state license plates they've seen on the trip, or the various tourist attractions they've visited. As you travel the road to becoming a nonsmoker, we strongly recommend that you also keep a journal. A small, 3" x 5" wirebound notebook will suit your purpose well. Such a notebook is about the size of a pack of cigarettes and can be placed easily into a shirt pocket or a purse, just where your pack of cigarettes formerly rested.

Substitute your journal for cigarettes

Use your journal as a substitute for your pack of cigarettes. Whenever you feel the need to reach for a cigarette, reach for your journal instead. Record your feelings of the moment. Keep your journal handy at all times. If you were in the habit of lighting up the moment your feet touched the floor in the morning, keep your journal on your bedside table at night. Instead of reaching for that first morning cigarette, reach for your journal. Write down how you are feeling.

Benefits of journal keeping

Although many experts have extolled the benefits of journal keeping, Morton T. Kelsey, in his book *Adventure Inward*, has said it especially well: "Keeping a journal can be of inestimable value in helping one sort through the difficulties, problems, and possibilities of life in order to manage one's life as well as possible. Few of us can hold together all the different threads of our lives unless we put them down one by one. It is strange how we can forget very important parts of our lives until we sit before a blank piece of paper and put them down one by one."[2]

Keeping a journal will be of invaluable assistance to you as you go through the quitting process. Your relationships with family and friends will be affected by your quitting process, as will your attitude toward work, home, and all of life. What was routine will become confusing. Just as in spring house or garage cleaning, you must choose what to keep and what to discard, so also in seeking a new nonsmoking life-style, you will be faced with the necessity of retaining some former concepts and beliefs about life and getting rid of others. You will need to relearn everything you do, learning to do it all as a nonsmoker rather than as a smoker—how to eat, drive, converse, cook, clean, etc.

Your journal will serve as a record of your quitting process and as a healing, therapeutic tool, helping you to view your smoking habit objectively. In it you will record your anxieties, stresses, and frustrations. Changing from a smoker's to a nonsmoker's life-style requires dealing with these anxieties, stresses, and frustrations. Over a period of time, as you reread what you have written, you will begin to observe patterns in your life. Your journal can be of considerable value in helping you sort out your difficulties and problems.

How to keep a journal

Begin your journal by introducing yourself and your smoking history. For example, My name is _____, and I have smoked for _____years, _____cigarettes, pipes, or cigars per day. Continue by listing all the reasons why you want to quit. Then list the reasons why you would like to continue smoking. Compile a list of alternatives to smoking. Such a list might include what to do, instead of smoking, while you sit at the dining room table and read the newspaper. (You might read the paper in a different room, or in an easy chair.)

When you quit smoking, you may experience several of the following physical symptoms: irritability, coughing, insomnia, dizziness, constant hunger, stomach cramps, constipation. Record your feelings of physical discomfort in your journal. As time passes and you reread these parts of your journal, you will see that these symptoms lessened and finally disappeared the longer you went without cigarettes.

Write about the anxiety, frustration, and anger you feel when you decide *not* to put that cigarette in your mouth. Write about your confusion as to who you are, now that you aren't smoking. Where do you fit into your world? What about all of those cigarette advertisements which feature beautiful, healthy-looking smokers? Where do *you* fit in now? Write about the insecurity you feel without your cigarettes. Write about your feelings of inadequacy in dealing with various people and situations without your cigarette in hand.

When being creative, we release many emotions. Morton Kelsey said, "When we live on top of an emotional volcano which is about to erupt, recording our feelings can help us move off it or even keep the explosion from occurring. Giving expression in the written word to the feelings which appear about to overwhelm and possess us often gives us distance from them. Then we begin to take control over our lives."[3]

Be sure to record the good feelings of quitting as well as the bad. Include a list of your successes: the first meal without a cigarette, the first coffee break, the first phone conversation, the first entire day without a cigarette. These are all significant process markers in your journey, worthy of a place in your journal. Here might be the spot to list your strengths and weaknesses, the beginning of building more self-confidence. Here, also, might be the place to start a food journal, a tool to help keep your weight under control.

Your journal will contain very personal, private communication, and therefore you may want to keep it away from other people. One friend of Morton Kelsey's, who teaches meditative prayer and journal keeping, passed on this request.

> Now I lay me down to sleep.
> I pray the Lord my soul to keep.
> If I should die before I wake,
> Throw my journal in the lake.[4]

If you have smoked for a long time, cigarettes have become your best friend—a friend who is always beside you, at your beck and call. When you quit smoking, that friend is gone. Write about how that makes you feel. Although your cigarette wasn't *truly* a friend, it felt like one. You may need time for actual mourning and healing. You may feel as though you have lost a part of yourself. Record those feelings.

Let God come more fully into your being. Let God replace the emptiness you feel at the loss of your cigarettes. God wants life for you, not death. When you take smoking out of your life, you may feel weak, but in this weakness is strength through the power of Jesus Christ (Phil. 4:13). Use your journal as the keeper of your feelings concerning the growing awareness of God acting and working in your life, of the love you are learning God has for you, and of the strength you can obtain through God.

Within your renewed faith, you will find courage to solve the complex problems of quitting smoking. You will find that as you conquer each problem, you will have the power to fulfill your unique God-given potential. You have always had the potential, but it has been dormant because you have let cigarettes take control of your life.

Now, take up your journal and organize a few goals around exercise, playtime, purpose of life, a support system in which you can express your feelings, and some form of daily relaxation. As you begin to change your life-style with these positive ways of dealing with stress, you will learn ways of dealing with your smoker-within. Remember to use deep breathing whenever you feel the urge to smoke. It provides a feeling similiar to that you associated with smoking.

Adjusting to Loss

*W*hen people experience a loss, they must come to grips with certain feelings. There is an entire grief process people must work through, whether the loss is a family member, a friend, a job, a home, or any other loss one might experience. When people quit smoking, a sense of loss also occurs.

Many people describe their cigarette as their "best friend." They tend to seek out this "best friend" in times of joy, anger, sadness, frustration, and so on, just as they would seek out a close friend to share thoughts and feelings with. It seems understandable, therefore, why you might experience a tremendous sense of loss when giving up your "best friend." In actuality, you experience an entire grief process, encompassing the five stages described by Elisabeth Kübler-Ross in her landmark book, *On Death and Dying*.[1]

DENIAL OR ISOLATION

The first stage in the grief process is called denial or isolation. When people find out they, or someone close to them, are dying their first reaction is often something like "This can't be true," or "I'll get another medical opinion," or "The tests must be wrong," or "Leave me alone. I don't want to talk about it." Common statements from smokers may be "I don't have a problem. I can play tennis or walk upstairs and never get short of breath," or "I can quit anytime," or "I have no family history of cancer or cardiovascular problems, and therefore I won't have a problem," or "Don't bug me about it. Leave me alone."

Mary Jo and Dick were married. She was a smoker. He was not. He tried hard to be tolerant of her habit but had a genuine concern for her health and would periodically try to discuss this with her. He was most often met with one of two responses from Mary Jo, either "I don't want to talk about it right now" *(isolation)*, or "I don't have a smoker's cough. I just have a little cold" *(denial)*.

ANGER

The second stage of the grief process is anger. Terminally ill people experience a sense of "why me?" This feeling is often accompanied by anger, resentment, even rage that this could be happening to them. A smoker's resentment comes out in, "Why do I have to quit smoking?" "Why does something I enjoy so much have to be so bad for me?" "I don't want to quit smoking; I enjoy smoking."

Ginny was taking part in a quit-smoking clinic and attended regular support group meetings following the clinic. One night at the meeting as the group was sharing, Ginny was overwhelmed by how easily everyone seemed to be coping with not smoking. For Ginny, every minute was a *struggle* not to smoke. Suddenly, she burst out,

"Why is it so easy for all you guys not to smoke and it's so hard for me?" Ginny was angry—angry that she ever smoked, angry that smoking was bad for her, angry that she had to quit, and angry that she liked smoking so much. Those feelings of anger and resentment are a normal, natural part of such a major life-style change.

BARGAINING

The third stage of the grief process, and one that most smokers are well acquainted with, is bargaining. This stage can be recognized among ill patients as they attempt to bargain with God for more time to complete this or that event in their life. For example, "Lord, let me live until my son graduates from school," or "Let us share one more Christmas together as a family." The smoker's bargaining possibilities are infinite: "I'll quit after Christmas," or "I'll quit after exams are over," or "I'll quit when my home life is nice and calm," and so forth. We all have important issues with which we bargain. Most smokers spend a lot of time bargaining as part of their process of quitting.

Carol said, "I was stuck in the bargaining stage for years. That's how I rationalized my smoking. I was always telling myself I would quit when the time was right. Then, I realized there was no 'right' time—just a time I chose to try."

Carol even rationalized about times when she might smoke again, a kind of bargaining. For example, at an advanced age one might say, "It wouldn't matter anyway."

DEPRESSION

The fourth stage is difficult and can be emotionally draining for many people. It is that of depression. When people who are dying begin to realize the inevitability of their own demise, they may want to spend much time alone and they may be quite tearful. Reality is setting in and their sense of loss is overwhelming. With people trying to quit smoking, depression is a normal and natural feeling. There is nothing wrong with tears. They may come freely at this time, and crying can be a very cleansing experience. Holding back the tears may even prolong this stage. Grief must be experienced—worked through—so that the smoker can let it go. After all, if your best friend died, you would feel tearful and sad, so why not over this "best friend"?

Sherry found herself crying easily and often when she was giving up cigarettes. For a while, she thought there was something wrong with her for "crying over a silly white stick." Then, she realized that she was saying good-bye to a friend, and the more she was able to talk about her feelings, the less depressed she felt.

ACCEPTANCE

The fifth stage is acceptance. At this point, dying patients make their wills and say their good-byes. They might say, "I've had a good life and I'm ready to go." It is a time of peace and tranquility. From smokers you might hear, "I stopped smoking. While it was hard to do, I stopped," or "It's hard, but that's OK. I can survive, even grow." This is the stage in which a good-bye letter (see pp. 71-72) to the cigarettes might be written, the stage in which you know what you must do even though it hurts. You may still want to smoke sometimes, but you choose consciously not to smoke.

Sam knew he was beginning to accept himself as a nonsmoker when he was offered a cigarette at a party and heard himself say, "No, thanks, I don't do that anymore." Inside he considered accepting the offer. He knew how to hold the cigarette, how good it would taste, and that he'd probably enjoy smoking it. But he made a conscious decision to say no because he was now a nonsmoker.

People do not necessarily go through these five stages in the order presented. They may go from one stage to another, on to still another, and then back again. For example, you might deny that smoking is harmful to your body one minute, bargain to quit in three weeks another minute, become angry because you know you should quit another minute, and go back to bargaining, saying you'll quit in a month. There is no set pattern. Every smoker experiences and works through this grief process in his or her own way.

Remember, it takes time to grieve. One of your major tasks will be identifying the various feelings that occur; another major task will be expressing these feelings to your support network of friends, family, co-workers, and quit-smoking support group. It is only through this verbalization that you will arrive, cleansed and comfortable, at acceptance.

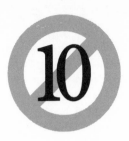

How to Handle Stress— without Smoking!

WHAT IS STRESS?

S tress. A most common word. We hear it used daily in reference to a multitude of things. Beginning a new job leads to stress, as does losing a job, having a baby, getting married or divorced, hitting a home run, striking out, or quitting smoking. Stress is a normal, daily part of life. Everyone experiences stress; different things cause varying degrees of stress. By definition, stress is the body's nonspecific response to any demand that is made upon it. Physically, stress can cause increases in the pulse rate, rate of breathing, blood pressure, the body's output of adrenalin, and it causes the body's immune system to be inhibited. When a person is exposed to prolonged high levels of stress without relief, great physical damage can occur. Emotionally, stress can cause irritability, depression, insomnia, and other symptoms. Smokers have an added risk because the nicotine in cigarettes produces many of the same effects (increased pulse, rate of breathing, and blood pressure), so a person smoking in response to stress adds insult to injury.

Stress has both positive and negative aspects. In the positive sense, stress is a powerful motivator for change. It fires us up when we have a big project to do, a paper to write, or some other difficult situation with which to cope. Without stress, we would not exist. On the negative side, stress may misdirect energy—causing distress—and may result in physical and psychological symptoms.

A smoker's usual response to stress is to light a cigarette. It might be that you believe smoking calms your nerves and helps you deal with stressful situations. Perhaps as you are working at quitting cigarettes, you are feeling the most stress you have ever felt. Giving up cigarettes may put you under tremendous stress for a time. Because cigarettes have been a part of your coping process for a long time, you may wonder how to deal with stress without cigarettes. Susie's son helped her find a way. Susie returned home from her stop-smoking retreat elated—she'd gone without cigarettes for several days! But she was also under a great deal of stress as she wondered how she would cope in the real world. That first evening home, when she went into the kitchen to prepare dinner, she found herself unable to coordinate thoughts and actions. Her 10-year-old son asked what was wrong and she responded, "I've never cooked dinner without smoking a cigarette, and I'm not sure I can do it." Her thoughtful son responded, "Sure you can! All you need is a hug!"

Before discussing healthier ways to cope with stress and stressful situations, let's look at the subject of health in general. For many years, medical science focused attention primarily on the treatment of illness and injury. In more recent years, however, the emphasis has switched to the area of prevention. Cost has been a big motivational factor as experts have discovered that with the rising cost of health care, it's less expensive to prevent illness than to treat it.

Illness and wellness are now looked at as a continuum, rather than as separate and distinct. At one end of the continuum is high level wellness; at the other end is premature death; in between are many varying levels of wellness.

When you stop smoking, you take a very big step along the wellness continuum, to a higher level of wellness. Likewise, when you identify causes of stress in your life and then learn positive, rather than self-abusive, ways to handle stress, you also take a giant step forward along this continuum toward a higher level of wellness. Self-education and growth in terms of smoking cessation and stress management are a big part of your progress.

Another important concept here is holistic medicine which is based on the fact that body, mind, and spirit must all be in good health for a person to be in a high level of wellness. In other words, if a person's body is disease free, but the person is depressed emotionally, that person is not very well. All three—mind, body, and spirit—function in relation to each other and influence each other.

HOW DO WE COPE WITH STRESS?

You've gone without a cigarette for two days. You bite your fingernails, can't sleep, snap at the people around you, and kick the refrigerator. You can't remember how to cook dinner, you're constipated, and you have a head-ache. Stress! How will you deal with it? Four ways to cope with stress are offered here.

Exercise

One way to deal with stress is to direct energy outward through exercise (see also pp. 72-73). Some type of daily exercise program is ideal, but a good start is three one-hour exercise periods per week. Your program may be as simple as an evening walk or as strenuous as two hours of tennis. The type of exercise you choose will undoubtedly depend on what you enjoy and how much exercise you are used to. Because everyone's interests and abilities are different, be sure to exercise only within your own limitations. Ask your doctor how much and what type of exercise would be best for you, based on your individual health history. You will find that the physical and psychological benefits of exercise are great.

When Mary quit smoking, her need for physical activity was so strong that she informed the people at home that she "had" to go running. For her, exercise wasn't even a decision; it was a strongly felt need that helped her cope with stress.

Playtime

A second way to deal with stress is with some type of compensation routine or playtime (see also p. 73). As children, we are encouraged by adults to concentrate, to be serious, to focus our attention. Many of us thus grow up to be serious adults who have totally forgotten how to play, relax, and have fun. We all need "time out," time purely for playtime, whether that be Frisbee, golf, curling up with a good book, or listening to classical music. Playtime may be needlework or model building or painting. Whatever it is, playtime can greatly reduce tension. The difference between playtime and exercise is a matter of attitude. For some people, tennis is exercise—

strenuous and competitive. For others, tennis is play-time—relaxing, noncompetitive, and conversational.

Joe found that he wanted his playtime to involve some intellectual stimulation. Though he was a lawyer by profession, he enrolled in a twice-a-week night class in photography, something he had always wanted to do. He was playing and having fun, yet substituting something enjoyable and healthy for his cigarettes—as well as coping with stress.

Express feelings

A third way to deal with stress is to express feelings. Smokers sometimes use cigarettes to keep a lid on feel-ings—to hold the feelings inside. As you begin to let go of your habit, feelings will begin to come out, and the more the better because expression of feelings reduces stress. Express feelings verbally, in writing, on a tape recorder, or in whatever way seems most comfortable to you. Dan, a young man who came to our stop-smoking clinic, found his cassette recorder to be an ideal tool for expressing his feelings. Whenever he became angry about something, he would go into the den, shut the door, and say what he was feeling on tape. After he verbalized his anger, he'd rewind the tape for the next time. The cassette provided a safe way for Dan to get rid of his pent-up anger and thus lower stress.

Take a look at your support network. Who are the significant people (family and friends) with whom you share thoughts and feelings? You need a support network of several people to listen to you as you work through feelings associated with giving up tobacco. Try to talk with others who are trying to quit, either individually or in a support group. Such people provide a great oppor-tunity to express feelings and may become an integral part of your support network. Remember that others cannot read your mind! If you want someone to know how you feel, you must tell them in clear and understandable terms.

"I" statements are more readily and easily heard than are "you" statements. Say, "I feel_____," rather than, "You make me feel_____." The listener is far more likely to be empathic to "I feel" than to "You make me feel. . . ." The accusatory "you" almost immediately elicits the defensive "not me," and any hope for hearing is lost.

The opportunity to talk about smoking and not smoking was tremendously important to Susie when she was quitting. She attended stop-smoking support group meetings for three months as this was a wonderful way to deal with the feelings accompanying smoking cessation.

Daily relaxation

A fourth stress reliever is a daily relaxation program which allows tension to flow from the body and provides both physical and psychological benefits. A relaxation program is, in essence, a form of mental hygiene. Although there are many different types of structured relaxation programs, simple deep breathing can have tremendous benefits in the early days of smoking cessation. This can be done inconspicuously, no matter where you are, and the tension relief is immediate. Two other types of relaxation programs are progressive relaxation, which focuses on tensing and relaxing various muscle groups, and autogenic relaxation, which focuses on the breathing process as a major support system.

The important point is that you choose a relaxation program that will help you to attain that state of relaxed internal awareness which is a prerequisite to achieving insight and growth. As you relax, your stress level will drop and your imagination, dreams, and visualizations will become clearer.

Visualization

The Simontons of the Cancer Counseling and Research Center in Fort Worth, Texas, have helped patients fight cancer with self-awareness techniques. They use relaxation and visualization techniques to help people participate in their own health and visualize their own recovery.[1]

Visualization, or imaging, can be a real aid to the individual's power and capacity for change and growth. All people function, to some extent, on visual cue. For example, an ex-smoker sees someone smoking and immediately thinks, "I want a cigarette." Through visualization we learn new responses to visual cues so that seeing someone smoking no longer elicits the desire for a cigarette but rather the reminder that we no longer smoke.

How does this work? Through repeated visualizations, we can actually retract patterns in the brain so that the same visual cue will elicit a different response. We image the original situation over and over, only with a different ending. For example, the Simontons' patients visualize over and over the cancer cells being destroyed in their bodies. In this same fashion, visualization can be used to give up smoking as the smoker visualizes him or herself in various situations *without* a cigarette in hand.

A world-class skier who was the victim of a terrible accident that left him a quadriplegic was once asked how on earth he managed to cope emotionally with the idea of never skiing again. His response was, "I go skiing every day." Visualization was his way of continuing to enjoy the sport he loved as well as coping with his new life-style.

Another way to look at the situation is in terms of internal and external reality. As we move out into the world, we face an infinite number of experiences and opportunities. There's a big, wide, wonderful world out there. What most people don't stop to realize is that, as we move into ourselves, we will discover an equally vast *internal reality.* It's like being confronted with a crisis and saying, "I'll never get through this." Then, at some point you do, and you look back and say, "Wow, I don't know how I did that." You got there by tapping that vast well of strength and courage that lies within all of us.

When we think of visualization, we might be reminded of Dwight Stone, the famous high jumper in the 1984 Olympics. As the TV cameras focused on his face, head nodding, everyone could see him visualizing in his mind's eye exactly how he would run and jump his race.

For many people, visualization may be a very religious experience as they commit themselves to the Holy Spirit for help and support. Prayer may become an integral part of the stop-smoking process before, during, or after visualization and may, in fact, be the single strongest source of support and encouragement.

The best way to begin to understand visualization is to experience a relaxation exercise, working through what we call a "guided image." Two guided images that work well are offered here.

Guided Image #1. Dim the room lights and sit in a comfortable position with arms and legs uncrossed. Ask a trusted friend or family member to quietly and slowly read you through the following steps or make a cassette tape of the commands and play it back for yourself. Caution the one who is reading to proceed very slowly and to repeat commands, keeping in mind that repetition is a big part of the power of visualization.

1. Close your eyes and begin to breathe slowly and deeply, relaxing after each exhalation.
2. Notice tension spots in your body, and, as you breathe, relax each spot.
3. Imagine that you are in a favorite place (beach, mountain, whatever). Note weather, sounds, smells, sights. Relax. Enjoy the place. Savor the environment.
4. As you relax in your special place, begin to consider the issue of quitting smoking.
5. Develop in your mind's eye a picture of the desire to smoke. Give it the characteristics of weakness and inadequacy. Slowly, begin to change the picture.
6. Now picture the "want to stop," the "desire to be a nonsmoker," to quit, to be free, to be cured. Begin to think of the characteristics of aggressiveness and power.
7. Now imagine the encounter between the "want to stop" and the "desire to smoke," with the "desire" being destroyed or eliminated from the body and the "want to stop" winning.
8. Slowly, open your eyes, stretch, relax.

Guided Image #2. Another guided image that is often effective is to mentally walk through a day with and without cigarettes. This exercise is begun just like guided image #1, with relaxing, breathing, and visiting a familiar spot (steps 1-3). Participants are then asked to relive a typical day in their life, remembering every cigarette they smoked. The leader walks them through the day, mentally (for example, remember breakfast: who was there, what did you eat, did you smoke, and so on). Then they are asked to relive the same day, this time with *no* cigarettes. Each activity is repeated, but without smoking. This image helps to prepare people for situations in which they may wish to smoke and it helps them to see other ways to handle these times. As people become more involved in themselves without cigarettes, it is also more likely that they will actually become nonsmokers.

After you have worked through these visualization processes it is important to discuss your experiences and share your feelings with others. One thing to keep in mind is that arrival is only an illusion. We never become perfect. Just when we think we have all the answers—that we have finally learned how to deal with all stress in our lives—we discover there's more to learn. And so it is with life; there will always be more to learn and do and grow, as long as we live. So, even though you may struggle to give up tobacco, remind yourself often that you are learning and growing and becoming a much stronger person. As you work through the quitting process, allow yourself to relax, visualize yourself as a nonsmoker, and keep stress under control.

Help! I'm Gaining Weight

You've quit smoking. You've finally joined the ranks of the nonsmokers. You are very proud of yourself. But your sweet victory is beginning to sour a bit as you watch the needle on your bathroom scale. The pounds are creeping on. You just *knew* this would happen. Many of your friends who have quit smoking complain of the same problem. Smoking, they claim, helped to keep their weight down, and when they quit, they gained. Are the extra pounds worth the trade-off? You value your slim body. Is the weight gain associated with quitting smoking a requirement, a necessary and inevitable by-product of kicking the habit?

We can shout a resounding "No!" but must also add, "Not if you are *extremely* careful." Although many smokers do gain a few pounds when they quit, an awareness of how and why this happens can prepare you as you work through the quitting process. And if you are prepared you can avoid most of those excess pounds.

WHY AM I GAINING WEIGHT?

The old belief that smokers gain weight when they quit smoking, simply because they eat more, is only partially true. Although many people do replace their cigarettes with candy, not everyone takes in enough calories from the extra food alone to warrant the weight gain. Some people are pleasantly surprised to find that their food seems to taste better when they haven't been smoking. And they may, therefore, tend to eat more.

Perhaps as you began the quitting process, you determined that you would *not* gain weight when you quit smoking. You would *not* trade one problem for another, and you were extremely careful to avoid overeating. You munched on celery sticks instead of candy. You practiced perhaps the best exercise of all—pushing yourself away from the table—but even after all your precaution you've gained a few pounds. What's the problem?

As with many problems, the causes for weight gain may be multifaceted. First of all, smoking and eating both provide oral gratification, which is our earliest and most practiced stress-reduction behavior! If we replace smoking with eating, we exchange one form of oral gratification for another. This may sound simplistic, but it is often true. We then have to ask ourselves if the extra pounds are worth the trade-off.

Sally had to ask herself this question as she gained 20 pounds after giving up smoking. Were those pounds worth not smoking? Two forces were at work here. One force was that of sabotaging herself or setting herself up to fail. If Sally gained weight, she would have an excuse to return to smoking. The other force was substituting the oral gratification of smoking with food. Whenever she wanted a cigarette, Sally went to the refrigerator for her "reward" (food).

Cigarette smoking has been labeled a negative addiction—something that provides instant gratification with long-term negative outcome. Alcohol addiction and food addiction fall within this same category, so don't get caught in choosing one negative addiction to replace another. Although many smokers do gain a few pounds when they quit, an awareness of how and why this happens can prepare you as you work through the quitting process. If you are prepared, you can avoid most of those excess pounds.

Another reason for weight gain in a person who has just quit smoking has to do with energy use and metabolism. When people smoke, they use energy. One of the metabolic responses to smoking is an increase in heart rate, with an increase in energy uptake or calories "burned." Think of the number of times you smoke each day. Simple mathematics says the number of cigarettes you smoke daily equals the number of times you increase the metabolic rate and calories burned. Take away that caloric "minus" and you see a decreased calorie need. In other words, a smoker who takes in 2000 calories per day will actually absorb only 1600 or 1700 calories. The nonsmoker's body will absorb the full impact of the 2000 calories. This is a surplus of 400 calories a day. There are 3500 calories in a pound, so in just nine days' time the new nonsmoker can easily gain a pound. This may not seem so bad, but when you think of that gain in terms of, say, nine weeks, it may add up to seven pounds or so—in just two months!

Still another reason for a weight gain after quitting is an enzymatic factor. In a lecture, John Maurer, M.D., explained that LPL (lipoprotein lipase), an enzyme that promotes fat storage, is found to be more "active" in smokers. When a person quits smoking, the transition time before LPL levels normalize to nonsmoker levels may result in added pounds.

These theories are just a few which help explain why people who are trying to quit smoking gain weight. But rather than bemoan these realities, most ex-smokers would rather hear tips to help them avoid weight gain. Here are a few.

TIPS TO AVOID WEIGHT GAIN

Examine your eating habits

Use your journal to record foods eaten, amounts, when, and mood at times of eating. Next, look for trouble spots—any time when you eat for reasons other than hunger. Ask: "Am I really hungry, or am I eating because I am bored, tired, or depressed? Have I begun to eat (instead of smoke) while I watch television? Am I using food as a tranquilizer for stress (whether it is the stress that accompanies quitting smoking or stress in other areas of my life)?" Once you've identified your problem areas, strategize to change behavior. Compile a list of alternative activities that will help to distract you from rampaging through the refrigerator!

Keep tempting foods out of the house

Or at least store them out of sight. For some of us, hunger is accentuated by the sight of tempting foods. If we don't see the food, we won't be motivated to eat.[1]

Get some exercise

Physical exercise is a distraction from eating and smoking. Not only will physical exercise distract you from smoking (or eating), it will induce calorie burning, thus counteracting the weight gain mentioned above. Exercise will contribute to the life-style change you need to make as you move from smoker to nonsmoker—as you begin to allow the nonsmoker within you to become stronger than the smoker. Exercise will also help improve your breathing, since increased air intake oxygenates your blood and cleans your lungs.

Change your environment

If it's not possible to dash out for exercise at the moment the urge to smoke or eat strikes, remove yourself at least mentally from your environment. Listen to music, read a book, get out of the kitchen, walk around your desk.

Avoid starving all day and eating one big meal

Eating only one big meal a day slows down metabolism. Plan to eat three meals a day, being sure to choose carefully the foods you eat at these three meals. Eat more carbohydrates and fewer fats and sugars. New findings suggest that eating carbohydrates triggers a greater increase in metabolism than does eating fats. If you eat foods such as fruit, potatoes, or rice, which seem to trigger less of the hunger-producing insulin, you will feel more content and satisfied. You will have less desire to snack. On the other hand, if you try to starve yourself, eating only one meal a day, you will surely one day go on that "big binge," and all your efforts will go down the drain.[2]

Behavior change is gradual. Set short-term daily eating guidelines. Chew your food slowly and avoid large portions. Acknowledge goal achievement with positive self-talk: "I practiced good eating habits today," or "I'll do even better tomorrow." If you need a snack, make it low calorie. Raw vegetables (without dips) and fresh fruits are excellent choices. Remind yourself daily that you *do* care about yourself and that you deserve the good things in life, such as nutritious food and a healthy body.

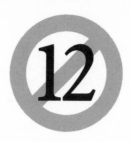

Dealing with Sabotage

When you hear the word *sabotage*, what kind of mental picture forms? Do you see a man, perhaps a spy, dressed in black, a cap pulled over his eyes, sneaking up on the enemy to dynamite their headquarters? Or do you imagine James Bond as he fights all the evil forces of the world? Such ideas about sabotage most likely were drawn from movies or television, which usually portray sabotage as sneaky, deceitful, and destructive action. Sabotage, however, is not limited to those media, nor is it a new concept. We see sabotage all around us in all areas of life and history, even as far back as Bible times.

The Bible contains numerous stories of people trying to interfere with the plans of others or trying to undermine various causes. Consider in particular a story from Genesis 37. Joseph, son of Jacob, shared with his brothers his dreams in which he appeared to rule over them. Jealous and fearful, the brothers threw him into a pit and then later sold him. The brothers wanted to get rid of the dreamer. They wanted to destroy him because they feared the power he might have over them. Their actions illustrate deliberate acts of sabotage, meant to put an end to what they considered to be frightening aspirations on Joseph's part.

Sabotage is all around us, functioning in numerous ways. As a new ex-smoker, you will certainly feel the old smoker-within (sometimes referred to as a *con*) trying to sabotage your new smoke-free life-style. One woman who quit smoking after coming to our church's stop-smoking retreat experienced a particularly heavy act of sabotage while on her first vacation as a nonsmoker. Lou's first thought when she and her husband stepped off the plane in the warm, sunny Caribbean was, "What a beautiful place not to smoke!" After a relaxing lunch in the hotel dining room, Lou excused herself to go to the restroom. On the way, she passed a cigarette machine. "Do you know," Lou told her stop-smoking support group later, "that machine tried to seduce me! It seemed to say, 'Come on, buy a pack!' " Lou ignored the machine and went on into the restroom. However, when she passed the machine again on her way back to her table, the temptation proved irresistible. Lou quickly pushed some coins into the slot, pulled the lever, grabbed the pack of menthol cigarettes that plopped out, and, like a guilty thief in the night, sneaked back into the restroom. Furtively, she slipped into a stall, and lit a cigarette. After a few drags, she came to her senses. *What in the world am I doing hiding in this stall, smoking menthol cigarettes—which I've always detested?* she thought. Furious with herself, Lou flushed the cigarettes down the toilet and returned to her table, grateful that the old sabotage trick had not completely ruined her resolve to be a nonsmoker.

Visualize a little con sitting on Lou's shoulder, calling attention to the cigarette machine and shouting, "I wanna smoke! I wanna smoke!" It's no surprise that Lou succumbed to such a temptation. Her con had waited until just the right moment and then attacked the new nonsmoker within Lou. A true act of sabotage! While Lou's smokeless life-style was sabotaged only briefly that time, sabotage can come—and come often—in many forms other than a cigarette machine. Thoughts such as, "Go ahead, one cigarette won't hurt," or "Reward yourself— you haven't smoked for 10 days," are sabotage. Below is a list of phrases that go along with the sabotage game.

Habit	I just found myself doing it. The first thing I knew, the cigarette was in my mouth.
Others Doing It	Everyone in my class smokes. Everyone was drinking and smoking.
Pleasure	I looked forward to that after-dinner cigarette. I really liked lighting up on a nice, spring day. I liked holding the cigarette and having the smoke in my mouth.
Craving	I began to feel itchy for a cigarette. I just couldn't wait to get a cigarette.
Anxiety	I got uptight and the cigarette helped me to relax. When I get upset, I want to reach for a cigarette.
Stimulation	I needed a quick lift.
Stimulus Control	I always smoked when studying. Smoking and drinking go together. At these business meetings, I always smoked.

Interestingly, the word *sabotage* originated from the French word *sabot*, meaning "wooden shoes." The story is told that many years ago in France, factory workers making *sabots* were unhappy with their working conditions. The workers tried to negotiate with management, but to no avail. In desperation, they threw their *sabots* into the machine, stopping production. Management was then forced to listen to the workers' problems.[1]

People trying to quit smoking are forced to deal with their con and with subtle outside forces as well. One gigantic force that has to be dealt with is that of the cigarette advertisments with their message that smoking provides happiness, attractiveness, sexuality, financial success, and a wonderful life-style. American cigarette manufacturers spend $1.5 billion a year on advertising in order to reinforce the idea that smoking is an "in thing" to do.[2] The tobacco companies make sure their messages are placed before the public at all times. For example, cigarette manufacturers often sponsor sporting events and virtually every sports stadium has at least one cigarette billboard. They also sponsor rock concerts and distribute free cigarettes. Through these and other marketing strategies, young people in particular are encouraged to become smokers.[3] What a force to sabotage the resolve not to smoke!

Other forces which sabotage new nonsmokers may include fear of managing one's life without the security of cigarettes, poor self-confidence, and the fear of change as they move from the easy familiarity of being a smoker to the potentially frightening "unknown" of being a nonsmoker.

You will need to work hard to move from smoker to nonsmoker. You'll need to pamper and analyze yourself constantly. You'll have to remember all those forces at work against you and learn to understand the sabotage games you will be tempted to play. You will have to remind yourself continuously that you don't smoke to stay slim, and that you might be cross and grouchy whether you smoke or don't smoke. If you can avoid the sabotage games listed earlier in this chapter, you will have come a long way toward your healthy, new life-style.

Tips to Help You Quit Smoking

*T*hroughout this book we have suggested a variety of tips to help you as you give up smoking. In this chapter we have consolidated these tips and added others that might help you withdraw from your habit. To aid you, we have broken the list of tips into three sections: physical, psychological, and spiritual. (You will note that some tips appear in more than one section.) We are aware that in order to be healthy you must be well in all areas. However, in order to accomplish this holistic task you might need to break down your problem areas, asking, "Are my physical symptoms getting me down? Are my psychological stresses putting me under? Have I placed my faith and trust in the Lord?" Think about your problem areas, analyze each, then choose the tips that will best help you quit.

DEALING WITH PHYSICAL WITHDRAWAL

Practice deep breathing. Breathe just as you do when you take a drag off a cigarette, only without the cigarette.

Deep breathing can be done in your car, at your desk, in a crowd, or wherever (Chapters 8 and 10).

Chew nicotine gum. It's a substitute for the drug, nicotine. Nicotine gum enables you to handle first the psychological and spiritual aspects of quitting smoking. Then, slowly, using the gum, you can withdraw from the physical aspects (Chapter 4).

Make goals to:

Exercise—it relieves stress and physical pain.

Play—it relieves stress and physical pain.

Verbalize—use your support system.

Meditate—take your problems to the Lord.

Set small, realistic stop-smoking goals.

Set a new direction for life.

(See Chapters 5, 8, 10, and 11.)

Other helpful hints include:

Drink plenty of water and fruit juices—oral gratification.

Eat vegetables and fruits—oral gratification and weight (Chapter 11).

Brush teeth often—oral gratification.

Chew gum, mints, or hard candy—oral gratification.

Take alternate hot and cold showers.

Get plenty of rest.

Alter regular behavior patterns. For example, take a new route to work; instead of sitting, go for a walk after meals; read the newspaper in a different chair; avoid cocktail parties or social situations; rearrange your household furnishings (Chapters 5, 6, and Appendix).

Get a new hairstyle.

Save the money you would have spent on smoking and reward yourself (Chapters 5 and 8).

Pursue a new hobby (Chapter 8).

Toy with a pencil, pen, or beads instead of a cigarette (Chapter 2).

Join an ongoing support group (see Appendix), or join an Alcoholics Anonymous support group.

DEALING WITH PSYCHOLOGICAL WITHDRAWAL

Take the "Why Do I Smoke?" test. This test will help you understand why you smoke (see Chapter 2).

Take the Myers-Briggs Type Indicator test to aid you in understanding your personality makeup and preferences (see the Appendix).

Confront your smoker-within by:
Taking personal responsibility.
Owning up to how much you smoke and why.
Understanding that quitting smoking is a process.
Desiring self-preservation.
Understanding that in order to become a nonsmoker, you must know your smoker-within (see Chapter 6).

Read over and over again the health risks to your body when you continue to smoke (see Chapter 4).

Keep a journal—a form of verbalization. This includes:
Writing a good-bye letter to your cigarette.
Making a list of reasons why you smoke.
Making a list of why you want to quit.
Making a list of your successes (see Chapter 8).

Build a new self, without smoking, by building new self-confidence (see Chapter 7).

Learn to cope with your negative stress by making new goals:
Exercise goals.
Play goals.
Goals about expressing feelings.
Goals for daily relaxation.
Goals for visualization (see Chapters 7 and 10).

For many people, giving up smoking is like giving up a good friend. When giving up this friend, most smokers go through a period of grief. Chapter 9 defines these various stages.

Be aware of the many games smokers play with their smoking, such as:

Smoking becomes a form of communication.

You live a certain kind of life-style when smoking.

Smoking can be used as a barrier in interpersonal relationships.

Smoking can be used to keep a lid on feelings.

Smoking can become a permission giver.

Smokers don't want to give up what is familiar or routine.

Smokers want to punish themselves.

Smokers are afraid of success without cigarettes (see Chapters 1 and 3).

Join an ongoing support group (see Appendix), or join an Alcoholics Anonymous support group.

STRENGTHENING SPIRITUAL GROWTH

Ask yourself, Have my cigarettes become an idol? (see Chapter 1).

Christians must be concerned with the stewardship of their bodies. Various themes throughout the Bible indicate the importance of the body. Read Genesis, Psalms, Leviticus, and John as examples (see Chapter 4). Life is a gift from God. Smoking promotes death (see Chapter 4).

Join a group:

Bible study group.

Prayer group (see Chapter 5).

Regularly ask God to help you quit smoking (see Chapter 5). Allow God to engage you:

Through a fellow Christian.

Through daily prayer.

Make goals to:

Meditate—take your problems to the Lord.

Change the direction of your life-style, asking God for
    guidance.

Help another person quit smoking.

Keep a journal. Record God's working in your life (see
Chapter 8).

Visualize your total surrender to the Holy Spirit for help
and support (see Chapter 10).

Join an ongoing support system (see Appendix), or join
an Alcoholics Anonymous support group.

Appendix

A Stop-Smoking Program for Churches, Businesses, Hospitals, and Communities

*T*he stop-smoking program designed and operated by Westminster and Eastminster Presbyterian churches in Grand Rapids, Michigan, has been in operation for 10 years. The initial concept of a retreat to help people stop smoking came from Westminster's senior pastor, Dr. John W. Stewart, himself a pipe smoker. The actual father of the program that followed that first retreat was also a pipe smoker—the Reverend Ray Kretzschmer, pastor of nurture and witness at Westminster Presbyterian Church. Marilyn Vander Veen has served the program since its inception as coordinator. Susie Heritage is director of lecturing.

Three retreats were held the first year. Evaluations of each retreat were extensive, providing impetus for change, growth, and problem solving so that the next retreats would be even better. Pastor Kretzschmer conducted training sessions for additional retreat leaders who were participants from the earliest retreats. As new non-smokers, they were ready to dedicate their time to helping others quit. Professionals, nurses and doctors, within the two churches' congregations stepped forward to offer their services. Church members gave encouragement, prayer support, and refreshments for retreats. *The Grand Rapids Press* and local television and radio stations provided free publicity for the stop-smoking program.

As people became convinced that smoking was, and is, detrimental to their health, and as they came to realize that smoking is no longer the "in" thing to do, the stop-smoking program grew. Currently eight to ten people serve as volunteer staff for the stop-smoking program. Each has dedicated time and skills to make a very successful program. Nearly all of the volunteers are former smokers, most of whom have quit through the stop-smoking program.

The stop-smoking program we use is not based on scare tactics or gimmicks but on education, nurture, and loving support. It is an excellent program for implementation in businesses, hospitals, and as a special ministry in churches. The following pages describe our program and can help you design a stop-smoking program for your group.

ORGANIZING A STOP-SMOKING PROGRAM

Our stop-smoking programs—retreats, clinics, and on-going support systems—are run entirely by volunteers. Over the years, these volunteers have been the major force in building the programs into what they are today, a caring, supportive method by which people can escape from nicotine addiction.

What we want to share here is how these volunteers wove their various skills into the foundation and building of these programs. It must be understood that most of the volunteers themselves had a need, a need to give up smoking. Ten years ago when the program first began, the structure was loosely organized. At that time, retreats were the only stop-smoking programs sponsored by the two Presbyterian churches and these were usually scheduled a year in advance.

Marilyn Vander Veen volunteered to coordinate the operation of the retreats; Rev. Ray Kretzschmer agreed to organize the lectures; various doctors from the churches volunteered to lecture on the physical aspects of quitting smoking. These were the beginnings of the organized structure. However, as the program advanced and clinics were formed and run in local businesses, colleges, and hospitals, a more organized structure was needed. More people who had quit smoking through retreats stepped forward to help, and volunteers and their unique skills were built into the program, and, in fact, became its very foundation. Based on our experience over the last 10 years, we recommend our stop-smoking program as a model for organizing yours.

Basically the structure is composed of a stop-smoking board, a director of the programs, and volunteers. Westminster Presbyterian Church has become our headquarters, providing office space, telephone, and supplies. Eastminster Presbyterian provides the campgrounds for the stop-smoking retreats. Following is a description of the function and responsibilities of volunteers used on our stop-smoking board, the director of the program, and the needs for other volunteers. (Our volunteers are from many different denominations.)

The stop-smoking board

The stop-smoking board is composed of:
- President
- Vice president
- Secretary/treasurer
- Personnel staff member
- Community awareness staff member
- Public relations staff member
- Other staff members (from the church, business, or community)
- Director of the stop-smoking programs
- Other volunteers (lecturers, doctors, psychologists, etc.)

The *president* oversees the entire board and programs. The president helps raise funds; fills in for lecturers; promotes good relationships with businesses, communities, colleges, and other churches; sets up program policies; directs future planning; and the like.

The *vice president* serves as liaison between the board and the director of the program. The vice president's most important function is to support the program director and to help solve any problems that arise in the programs.

The *secretary/treasurer* keeps records and pays expenses. This entails setting up a checking account and having a computer available. A computer has been available for our use since the beginning of our program; names and addresses of all the participants from the last 10 years are on a disk. We have also recorded on a disk all correspondence and financial records.

The *personnel staff member* assists in finding the program director. (If any one position might *not* be volunteer, but a paid position, it would the director of the programs.)

The *community awareness* staff member helps make program policies and raise funds, and serves as a liaison between our programs and the communities, churches, businesses, and others.

The *public relations* staff member organizes publicity for all the programs.

Other staff members are church staff, session representatives, personnel directors, commissioners, and so forth.

The *director of the stop-smoking programs* is responsible for the operation of all the stop-smoking programs. She or he organizes the skills of the volunteers and sets the schedule for the retreats, clinics, and support groups. The director negotiates with the hospitals, businesses, communities, or churches whenever and wherever programs are held.

Volunteers should be asked to be on the board according to need. For example, if you are just starting to run a stop-smoking program, you will want to ask a doctor and a psychologist to be on your board. The doctor will lecture on physical health and the psychologist will train other volunteers in organizing their lectures.

We ask board members to serve for three years. At the end of that time they may continue to serve or be replaced by another volunteer. When necessary, the president of the board selects a small group of volunteers to choose replacements when board members leave.

Volunteers

As stated previously, volunteers are the foundation for the stop-smoking program. Listed below are some of the needs of the stop-smoking program and how these needs were filled by volunteers in our programs.

Publicity: Margie Dawe arranged to have our retreats advertised on the backs of city buses. Mary Ann Schumaker, an artist, made posters that were placed throughout the city. Ann Kutzli suggested these possibilities for free advertisements about a stop-smoking program.

- Free publicity is available to all nonprofit organizations through radio and television stations and newspapers.
- Talk with radio and television stations to determine public service policy.
- Talk with local newspapers about a feature article.
- Talk with the mayor since city or town offices may be willing to announce something like a "nonsmoker's week" or a "stop-smoking day." Make it official and gain some publicity through a news conference.
- Ask other churches to announce the date of your program through their bulletins.

Lecturers: Susie Heritage, a professional nurse who had trained other nurses, organizes and lectures on topics such as stress and the grief process. Sue Taylor, who works with arthritic patients in a local hospital, lectures on responsibility. Dennis Wales, salesman, lectures on keeping a journal. Dr. John Stewart, senior pastor at Westminster Presbyterian Church, lectures on motivation and ways to quit. These are examples of some of our lecturers. All of these people have a background in communication and have been trained in listening and speaking skills (see pp. 118-121).

Here are some of our other volunteers. Bill Esch is the *cook* for the retreats; he has battled many serious and prolonged problems with his own health. *Housemother* for the retreats is Dana Ziebarth who helps participants feel at ease. Some other workers at the retreats are Chuck

LeBlanc who quit a five-pack-a-day habit at a retreat and who is a source of inspiration to many other people; Jim Sailors who sold himself on the concept of quitting and is now selling others on the same concept; Donna Bonney who brings the gift of listening to others trying to quit; Lenore Dunn who likes to share her story of quitting and who often helps in the kitchen. We also have volunteers to lead sports events, exercise time, the worship service, to clean the retreat center, and the like. *Support* is led by Mary Ippel who is skilled in listening and Dick Thorne who shares himself in order to support other people. The *doctor* at our events might be Dr. John Maurer, Dr. William Cayce, Dr. Paul Clodfelder, or Dr. Bert Dugan who give freely of their time toward this ministry.

We have seen the corps of volunteers in our program as one body with many different members. Paul told the Corinthian church (1 Cor. 12:1-13) that they were composed of many different members with many different gifts, and the same is true of the stop-smoking program. Our volunteers have come with a variety of gifts. It takes many gifts to make the programs run; any one person or any one gift alone isn't enough. Many people must share their gifts in order for the program to be a success. All these gifts together is what volunteerism is all about, tapping each resource for individual abilities and then pulling them all together.

As you begin a similar stop-smoking program in your church, community, or business place, you will want to seek out volunteers to help set up and design the program. Former smokers are, of course, preferable to people who have never smoked. After your first clinic, retreat, or ongoing support system, you will most likely be able to draw new volunteers to help with your programs—people who have successfully moved through the program, people who have "been there" and are now gratefully willing to help other smokers quit.

While the talents and abilities you'll find in your volunteers are a wonderful resource, providing some educational opportunities to supplement those talents can make them even more effective. Excited, willing volunteers with their own unique gifts can become even more valuable if they receive some additional training. Such training might include:

- Attending a clinic, retreat, or a few weeks at an ongoing support group—not as a participant, but for the sole purpose of learning firsthand how a clinic, retreat, or support group is run.
- Training sessions on listening skills.
- Training sessions on public speaking.

Below you will find additional information on listening and speaking skills.

Listening skills. Nancy Clodfelder, a trainer for the Amity listening skills, says that listening is a gift. Listening is a sign that you care. It is a prime way to show nonjudgmental acceptance. Listening to another person is an act of giving yourself to that person, while creating a trust relationship.[1] During training sessions for those people who will work with persons who are trying to stop smoking, listening skills need to be highly emphasized. Listening to someone who is trying to give up a part of their identity takes patience and practice.

Volunteers working with people who are trying to quit smoking need to be exceptionally good listeners. Smokers who take the courageous step of coming to a stop-smoking retreat or clinic must trust that they will be heard, that they will be listened to. They must believe that the one listening will sympathetically take in all that they say: all their anger, struggling, and anxiety. Smokers who are trying to quit need to talk about the pain they are feeling. They must know that the volunteer *feels* their pain, *understands* their pain.

What is listening? We know we do it with our ears; we know we listen more than we speak; we know it takes real work to be an effective listener. Todd Oleson, psychiatric social worker at Holland Community Hospital in Holland, Michigan, says there are many definitions, thoughts, and ideas about listening, ranging from the "folksy" and simple to the technical and complex. Listening has been called love . . . creativity, the other side of talking.

Listening begins early. Human beings learn to listen before they speak, read, or write. Listening is the main channel for instructions, making up 45 percent of our daily communications. With the increasing significance of the mass media in our lives, the importance of listening rises. All of our thinking—our concepts—religious to economic, political ideals, ethical standards—are increasingly influenced by what we hear through radio, TV, and tape.

Listening is not done just with the mind, but with the entire body. What you do with your physical self while you are listening has a powerful effect on the other person. For example, take notice of the nonverbal signals you give when you are listening to someone. Is your body in a relaxed but attentive position? Are you making regular eye contact? Do your facial expressions reflect your own or other's feelings? Are you giving your full attention to listening? According to Amity, effective nonverbal skills (1) are comfortable for talker and listener; (2) help you listen and remember; (3) communicate interest and respect; and (4) increase the talker's feelings of trust and self-worth.[2]

Your volunteers will, at some point, share their own stop-smoking stories. They need, however, to be careful not to be too anxious to tell their own stories but to be ready to listen to others'. Volunteers may be so anxious to help—to "solve the problem"—that they may talk too much and miss what the other person is really trying to say. The very nature of humans is to be problem solvers. People trying to quit smoking, however, need a sounding board more than they need a problem solver.

Active listening is a learned skill requiring practice. Clodfelder says that the training session on communication or listening skills is very basic, but it does give people who are trying to help others quit smoking another tool in order to be more effective. Most of the people that are in the helping arena are already very good listeners because they care for other people and their feelings. The techniques emphasized help to enhance those qualities.

Speaking skills. The lecture is a large part of the stop-smoking program. Lectures are usually given by volunteers, all of whom should be trained as effective speakers. Oleson defines *lecture* as the orderly treatment of a particular subject for the purpose of instruction. We recommend the following four general guidelines for speakers.[3]

1. Be specific and concrete. Communication is hampered by vague generalities. Consolidate the material and convey the message in the most efficient manner possible.

2. Consider your listeners' frames of reference. Consider your listeners' backgrounds, intelligence, attitudes, and so forth, so that you can put the lecture in terms that they can understand. In particular, try to avoid "talking over the heads of your audience" and steer clear of jargon or special terminology that is foreign to your listeners.

Try to illustrate your ideas with examples that your listeners will be able to relate to on the basis of their experiences. The people in your stop-smoking group will have a short listening span, not to mention an abundance of anxiety, anger, fear, and frustration. It will be important to practice your lecture at home, testing yourself on a tape recorder or to a friend. Time yourself and notice weak spots.

Illustrations with examples are necessary to help keep the audience listening. For example, use handouts, use the chalkboard, and try the puppet show (see pp. 150-152).

3. Avoid "loaded" words. Certain words are loaded in the sense that they tend to trigger emotional reactions. In the interests of effective discourse, it is usually best to avoid using such words as *can't* and *should*. Such words may bring on feelings of helplessness and guilt.

4. Make your verbal and nonverbal messages consistent. When you give a lecture, make sure your nonverbal messages match your words (your facial expressions, eye contact, postural variations, and touch). For example, it would be unwise to lecture on the importance of keeping a journal while yawning and slouched in a chair, eyes half closed. Be consistent, both verbally and nonverbally.

Your program's volunteers will be able to draw much of the information for their lectures from this book. This material, of course, needs to be combined with their own experiences and any additional resources available. All volunteers should plan their lectures carefully.

RETREATS, CLINICS, AND ONGOING SUPPORT SYSTEMS

We began our stop-smoking program with retreats and eventually added six-session clinics as an alternative to the retreats. The clinics are designed especially for those who are unable to get away for an entire weekend, or who prefer the clinic over the retreat structure.

A few years later, in response to the needs of people struggling to remain nonsmokers and even to some who had relapsed (gone back to smoking), we implemented an ongoing support system. As you explore the idea of beginning a stop-smoking program in your church, business place, or community, you may choose to use the retreat, clinic, or support group structure. All three of them are currently in use in our stop-smoking program.

Statistics tell us that 47 million Americans use tobacco in the form of cigarettes and that cigarettes cause more illness and death than all other drugs.[4] Smoking *is* a problem in the U.S.! The programs at Westminster and Eastminster Presbyterian churches began in response to a need—people who were desperately seeking help to withdraw from nicotine addiction. Whether you view your decision to begin a similar program as a ministry in your church or as a service to your co-workers or community, perhaps even to your employees, you can rest assured that you will be meeting a desperate need.

People from every place in life are trying to quit smoking. Smoking is much less the "in" thing to do than it was years ago. Many people who puffed contentedly for years are now trying to quit. Smokers are finding more and more restrictions placed on *where* they may smoke as "no smoking" signs are being placed in businesses, schools, and retail stores. Most restaurants have designated seating areas for smokers and a few have even banned smoking entirely. More and more manufacturing plants and educational institutions are restricting smoking to specifically designated areas. Smokers are being told that not only are they playing Russian roulette with their own health, but that they are jeopardizing the health of nonsmokers who suffer from burning eyes, sore throats, and breathing problems that they may incur just from breathing smoke from someone else's cigarettes. Smokers in more and more situations are not in the majority but are "odd-person-out." While many smokers ignore all the hullabaloo, many more are taking it seriously and are making an effort to quit. In the last few years, government statistics tell us approximately 10 million people have kicked the habit. Still other statistics tell us that many people fail or go back to smoking. It is at this point that stop-smoking programs can be of invaluable assistance.

If you are interested in implementing one of these programs in your church, business place, or community, see the section on organizing a stop-smoking program (pp. 112-121).

Retreats

The weekend retreat structure for quitting smoking offers a haven away from the stress of our busy world; a quiet place where people can meditate, enjoy nature, and take a complete break from cigarettes. At a retreat there are no spouses, children, jobs, or telephones. And smoking is not allowed. We have found that a church camp or retreat center provides a perfect place for conducting the stop-smoking retreats.

While for many people quitting smoking is a long, slow process, for some it is an *abrupt break* from tobacco use. Dr. John W. Stewart, senior pastor of Westminster Presbyterian Church, says, "People need an opportunity to stop-smoking 'cold turkey' but within a context of encouragement and acceptance over a period of a few days. Behavior adjustments require a sense of internal dissonance, a willingness to change, and a supportive corporate experience. Retreats are an appropriate setting for such a change in human addiction."

The retreat then provides this atmosphere. Because smoking is not allowed during a retreat, a complete break from cigarettes is necessary. Even though a person goes without cigarettes for three days, she has not totally succeeded in becoming a nonsmoker, because at this point the smoker within is still much stronger than the nonsmoker. That is why an ongoing support system is necessary for those who choose the retreat method, as well as for those who "quit" over a longer period of time. Life-style changes are necessary for all people who wish to become nonsmokers.

We recommend the following objectives, suggestions, supplies and materials, and schedule for a stop-smoking retreat.

Objectives

1. To assist participants in exploring the issue of stopping smoking.
2. To look at smoking within the context of wellness on all levels.
3. To educate participants about smoking issues, equipping them personally to examine the issue.
4. To introduce "working tools" participants may choose to use to assist themselves.
5. To assist in the establishment of a functioning support group within the community or to assist participants in joining an ongoing support system. (See pp. 139-149 for information on forming an ongoing support group.)

Suggestions

1. The best group size is 13 to 18 people. We suggest that there be no *more* than 20 but no less than 10 people per retreat.
2. The retreat should be held on a weekend, beginning at noon on Friday and ending at approximately 5:00 P.M. on Sunday.
3. A support group should be formed immediately following the retreat (for those who cannot use the ongoing support groups), or suggest that each participant join an already established support group.
4. A nominal fee should be charged to cover retreat expenses.

Supplies and materials

Food for 2 breakfasts, 2 lunches, 3 dinners, and for snacks.

We chart our menus on paper so that when purchasing food, we have a consolidated list of groceries to purchase. We try to select foods that most people like and we always have plenty of raw vegetables, fruit, and juices available as substitutes for cigarettes.

Program materials needed include: a folder for each participant containing an application form, a 3″ x 5″ spiral notebook, the "Why Do You Smoke?" test (see Chapter 2), a copy of the agenda, an outline of each lecture, handouts such as "A Guide to Quitting Smoking" from the U.S. Department of Health and Human Services, "The Way We Eat" from the Rhode Island Department of Health, The Clean Indoor Air Act—Public Act #198, descriptions of relaxation techniques, and various photocopies of articles pertaining to smoking from newspapers or magazines.

Other supplies and materials: movies or tapes and projection equipment, name tags, chalkboard and chalk, magazines for casual reading, extra pencils, games to play after evening lectures, equipment to be used for the Saturday afternoon free time.

Schedule

Friday

Tasks

To build a community.
To establish a trust between lecturers and participants and among the participants.
To give tools to smokers to help them quit.
To assist the participants in understanding the smoker-within.

Activities

12:00   People arrive and get settled. Lunch is served. People are entering a strange place, with people they don't know and without their cigarettes. They will be uneasy. Plan something for them to do after they are settled. You might ask for aid in food preparation, such as cleaning fruit and vegetables. Be sure to provide a variety of magazines and books that participants might pick up and read. Volunteers should meet each person at the door and give them a name tag and a folder containing the items listed above. They should then show them where to put their suitcases and bedding.

(Have plenty of volunteers available at this time.) During lunch, the volunteers should make light, easy conversation with the participants. (It might be the first lunch without smoking for some participants.) Because the volunteers understand what the participants are going through, a warm, caring community begins to form. As the volunteers share their stories of giving up smoking, the participants will begin to relax and feel at ease.

1:30   Welcome. The welcome is given by the retreat coordinator who introduces herself and the other retreat staff members. As retreat coordinator, be sure to praise participants for taking such a big step toward becoming a nonsmoker by coming to the retreat.

Explain that there will be no scare tactics or gimmicks used but that staff members, themselves all former smokers, are there to nurture, educate, and support. Reassure participants that they *can* quit smoking and that by doing so they will not only be doing themselves a favor healthwise, but also in terms of creating for themselves an exciting, new smoke-free life-style.

Be sure to emphasize that no smoking is allowed on the retreat.

Assign participants their "K.P." times.

Next, share your own stop-smoking story.

Introduce the concept of goal setting and keeping a journal (see Chapter 8).

Briefly go over the folder items. Provide time for participants to complete the "Why Do You Smoke?" test.

4:00   Encourage participants to relax by introducing some deep-breathing exercises.

4:30   Free time: Suggest that participants take a walk—a good substitute for smoking.

(You will note that we have not yet asked the participants to share their names or smoking histories. We have done this for a reason. During the first few hours of the program, most participants are defiant about their smoking habits. We break down this defiance by telling our story of quitting and by establishing a warm community. By the evening session most participants are eager to share their smoking histories.)

6:00   Dinner.

7:30   Lecture, "Your Smoker-Within" (see Chapter 6), to be given by a staff member.

Ask several staff members to share briefly their own stop-smoking stories.

Next, ask participants to pair off. Instruct them to spend the next 15 to 20 minutes interviewing each other, using the following discussion-starter questions written out on the chalkboard.

a. How many cigarettes do you smoke each day?

b. Why do you want to quit?

c. How long have you smoked?

d. Have you tried to quit before?

e. What will be the hardest cigarettes to give up (for example, those smoked after meals, those smoked on coffee break)?

f. Are there any unusual circumstances involved in your smoking?

After the interviewing, the group reassembles and each person introduces the person whom they have just interviewed and shares the personal smoking history of that person. This exercise enhances the community-building process. The lecturer who spoke earlier moderates this sharing time, being sure not to try to solve problems at this point, but encouraging participants to look for ways in which to solve their own problems. The lecturer should remind people that just as their smoking histories are unique, so also will be their quitting process. There is no one way to quit. Some people choose to quit "cold turkey" and some go three weeks without a cigarette, smoke one, and must begin the quitting process all over again.

Be sure to empathize with the participants. Remember that they are hurting. Spend some time explaining the necessity of their relearning or changing their routines, both on the retreat and when they return home. Tell them that they may need to take a different route to work, eat different foods, get up from the table after eating and take a walk (rather than smoking a cigarette), find a new hobby, do something they've never done before, listen to tapes or chew on carrots, celery, or straws while driving, and so forth.

Emphasize journal keeping, reminding participants to substitute their journal for cigarettes. The journal can serve as an emotional release; it can become a friend. Also encourage participants to get plenty of exercise.

As staff members share and empathize with participants, trust will develop and sharing among participants and leaders will become easier and more open. As leaders convey their awareness of the pain that the participants are going through, a natural, built-in mechanism seems to emerge—that of a former smoker compelled to help a smoker to quit.

End Friday with some kind of "light" activity, such as a humorous movie (serve popcorn and soda pop), games, storytelling, or television. Remember, plenty of rest is necessary for people who are trying to quit smoking. The retreat center should provide a comfortable place for rest, exercise, and relaxation. Meals should be nutritious and well-balanced.

Saturday

Tasks

To continue community building.
To encourage participants to evaluate the smoker-within.
To provide tools to help smokers as they go through the quitting process.

Activities

8:00	Jog or walk.
8:30	Exercise and shower.
9:00	Breakfast.
9:30	Lecture on the five principles of change (see Chapter 5).
10:00	Free time (a good time for leaders to take a walk with and/or talk with participants on a one-to-one basis).
12:00	Lunch.
1:00	Lecture on building self-confidence (see Chapter 7).
	Sharing time.
	Lecture on sabotage (see Chapter 12).
	For the remaining time before dinner, plan some kind of activity in which the group can act as a unit. For example, use the goal-setting ideas about play (see p. 73) or enjoy some kind of activity such as tennis, swimming, or softball. Encourage participants to help decide how the group will spend this play time.
6:00	Dinner.
7:00	Doctor's lecture. Information for such a lecture is included in Chapter 4. You may choose to invite a doctor from your church, local hospital, or community to speak to the group.
	After the doctor's lecture, allow free time for a movie, discussion, or exercise.

Sunday

Tasks

To continue community building.

To continue to evaluate the smoker-within.
To provide more tools to help smokers as they go through the quitting process.

Activities

8:00	Jog or walk.
8:30	Exercise and showers.
9:00	Breakfast.
10:00	Worship service. Invite a pastor (preferably a pastor who smoked and quit) or ask one of your volunteers to lead the worship service. One of the most meaningful worship services we had was when a participant shared how she quit smoking and how God played a major role in that process. Include music in the service; it provides wonderful therapy, and share plenty of hugs!
12:00	Dinner (save dessert for later).
1:00	Lecture on stress, relaxation, and visualization (see Chapter 10).

Next, allow time for people to discuss their fears about going home—about leaving the haven of the retreat center and re-entering the real world. Allow participants to share their fears. End this time by asking people to write a good-bye letter to their cigarettes (see pp. 71-72).

3:00	Coffee and dessert.
3:30	Distribute evaluation forms (see sample, p. 153).

Lecture on theory of loss (see Chapter 9). Allow time after this lecture for people to discuss how they are feeling. At this point, encourage reflection on changes they'll have to make in their lives if they are to allow the nonsmoker within themselves to become larger than the smoker-within. (People now should have gone three days without a cigarette and the group has become a community. Sharing their loss with each other will be very meaningful. Sharing new goals will also be important.)

End the afternoon by outlining the necessity and function of the ongoing support group. Explain how the group works and when it will meet and related matters (see pp. 139-149 for more information about support groups).

Award certificates. Sample wording: Certificate of Success and Honor. (Person's name) has begun the process of quitting smoking by successfully completing a non-smoking clinic. (Signatures, place, date.)

5:00 Say good-bye and leave for home.

As the participants leave for their homes on Sunday afternoon, a sense of peace should prevail. They know they are part of a community, all members of which are fighting the same battle. The sense of belonging, of being listened to and cared about, should have been firmly implanted at the retreat.

For the staff, the retreat provides a place to share the love of God and to give of themselves. David Myers, author of *The Human Puzzle,* says: "Biblical and psychological perspectives both remind us that faith is like love: if we hoard it, it will shrivel; if we use it and give it away, we will have it more abundantly. And that's the way it is with all God's gifts."[5]

Clinics

In stop-smoking clinics smokers meet for 1½ hours each day for six days (probably evening sessions), then enter the ongoing support system. The goal of the clinic is to build community, identify problems associated with quitting, and provide support for those who are struggling.

Clinics may be offered through businesses, hospitals, and churches for people who have a limited amount of time available for a stop-smoking program, or who perhaps have family, work, or school obligations on weekends which they cannot reschedule to allow for an entire weekend away. Our clinics are held in local hospitals, in churches, and in business places.

We recommend the following objectives, suggestions, supplies and materials, and schedule for a stop-smoking clinic.

Objectives

1. To assist participants in exploring the issue of stopping smoking.
2. To look at smoking within the context of wellness on all levels.
3. To educate participants about smoking issues, equipping them personally to examine the issue.
4. To introduce "working tools" participants may choose to use to assist themselves.
5. To assist in the establishment of a functioning support group within the community or to assist participants in joining ongoing support groups. (For information on forming an ongoing support group, see pp. 139-149.)

Suggestions

1. The best group size is 13 to 18 people. We suggest that there by no *more* than 20 but no *less* than 10 people per clinic.
2. The clinic should be held for six days, Monday through Friday, and the following Monday. Each meeting should last 1½ hours, the time to be selected by the community.
3. A support system should be established, or suggest that each participant join the already established support system.
4. A nominal fee should be charged to the participants.

Supplies and materials

Program materials needed include: a folder for each participant containing an application form, a 3″ x 5″ spiral notebook, the "Why Do You Smoke?" test (see Chapter 2), a copy of the agenda, an outline of each lecture, handouts such as "A Guide to Quitting Smoking" from the U.S. Department of Health and Human Services, "The Way We Eat" from the Rhode Island Department of Health, The Clean Indoor Air Act—Public Act #198, descriptions of relaxation techniques, and various photocopies of articles pertaining to smoking from newspapers or magazines.
Other supplies and materials: name tags, chalkboard and chalk, extra pencils.

Schedule

Monday

Tasks

To build a community.

To establish a trust between lecturers and participants, and among the participants.

To assist the participants in understanding the smoker-within.

Activities

Each participant is met at the door by a volunteer and is given a name tag and a folder which contains the items listed above. In the folder is an application which the participant is asked to fill out.

First lecturer—

1. Welcome. The welcome is given by a lecturer who introduces her- or himself, outlines the clinic agenda, and tells her or his personal stop-smoking story. This evening's lecturer should be sure to praise participants for their courage in coming to this meeting—for taking this first big step toward wellness.
2. Introduce the concept of goal setting and keeping a journal (see Chapter 8).

Second lecturer—

1. Welcome participants. Introduce yourself and share your smoking history.
2. Emphasize that no smoking will be allowed during meetings.
3. Give lecture on "Your Smoker-Within" and the five principles of change (see Chapters 5 and 6).

Both lecturers—

Ask each person to complete the "Why Do You Smoke?" test (in folder). Talk about the test and then allow each person an opportunity to speak and perhaps to share a few words about themselves.

Tuesday

Tasks

To continue community building.
To help smokers understand the smoker-within.

Activities

The entire meeting is dedicated to smokers sharing their smoking histories. Ask participants to pair off. Instruct them to spend the next 15 to 20 minutes interviewing each other, using the discussion-starter questions from pp. 128-129 (retreat schedule). After the interviewing, follow the suggestions given in the retreat schedule.

As lecturers share and empathize with participants, trust will develop and sharing among leaders and participants will become easier and more open. As leaders convey their awareness of the pain that the participants are going through, a natural, built-in mechanism seems to emerge—that of a former smoker compelled to help a smoker to quit.

Wednesday

Tasks

To discuss physical problems associated with smoking.
To help smokers understand the smoker-within (habit).

Activities

Allow the first half hour of the meeting for sharing, making sure that each participant has a chance to be heard.

Invite a doctor to lecture on the health aspects of smoking. Information for such a lecture is included in

Chapter 4. You may choose to invite a doctor from your church, local hospital, or community to speak to the group.

Thursday

Tasks

To understand the smoker-within (stress).
To identify creative ways of alleviating stress.

Activities

Present lecture on stress, relaxation, and visualization (see Chapter 10). Use the guided images (also included in Chapter 10, pp. 93-95).

Friday

Tasks

To understand the smoker-within.
To describe the five stages of the grief process.
To prepare for the weekend by looking at how smokers sabotage themselves.

Activities

1. Allow the first half hour for sharing, making sure that each participant has a chance to be heard.
2. Present lecture on theory of loss (Chapter 9).
3. Present lecture on sabotage (Chapter 12).
4. Ask participants to split up into two groups and to talk about which are the hardest cigarettes for them to give up (after meals, with coffee, etc.) and what fears they

have about getting through the weekend ahead without a cigarette.

Second Monday

Tasks

To understand the smoker-within.
To recognize themselves as authority in their lives.
To set goals.
To set up a support system.
To evaluate the clinic (see sample, p. 153).
To receive certificates.

Activities

1. Allow the first half hour for sharing, making sure that each participant has a chance to be heard.
2. Present the material on building self-confidence (see Chapter 7).
3. Let each individual talk about the personal goals they have set up to help alleviate stress during the coming weeks.
4. Distribute evaluation forms and provide time for completing them.
5. Award certificates.
6. Explain the ongoing support system.

Ongoing support systems

Joining a support system is important when you give up your smoking habit. For example, we learned in Chapter 5 in the section about joining a group that a support group provides a place where you share your weaknesses, receive praise for your successes, and are held accountable.

In dealing with the problems of giving up a habit, whether it be addiction to smoking, alcohol, food, or something else, it helps to know that you are not alone in your struggles—that others are going through the same thing. It helps to know that you can use each other as sounding boards or that you can air your problems with another person.

Finding the needs. We organized our ongoing support groups after studying the needs of the people who attended our clinics and retreats. We found that if the participants had a place every week to share their difficulties in giving up smoking, they were more apt to quit permanently. If we could get them to share their anger, additional stresses, or self-image problems with the group, the participants could then begin to deal with these problems. The Myers-Briggs Type Indicator test helped us determine still another need for the support system: those participants who lived by a schedule used the support group as a way to set up a new schedule.

In addition to studying the needs of our own people, we researched the smoking issue at a large university. This research indicated that many people relapsed or returned to smoking after a brief time of quitting. Interestingly, the research did not indicate *why* people returned to smoking, only that many people *do* relapse. We felt that this group of people might be able to use a support group as the place to start their process of quitting smoking all over again.

There was still one other group of people we felt might benefit from a support system. They are the people who might be tempted to return to smoking after having quit for a long time, perhaps even years. For example, when an ex-smoker is faced with a crisis, the first thing he or she wants to do is smoke. If, however, a support group is available for the ex-smoker to share this crisis, then the group can become a release instead of the cigarette.

Organizing the support group. We saw a need and decided to implement an ongoing support system. This was only the beginning, however. Next came the questions about how to structure the support group. For example, what kind of training did our volunteers need in order to lead the support groups? What size should the group be? Where should we hold our meetings? How should we structure meetings? After identifying the questions, we began to look for answers. We began first by looking at how we might train our volunteers. Rev. Ray Kretzschmer pointed out the two most important skills needed for volunteers who would lead support groups: a knowledge of group dynamics and good listening skills. He recommended a manual, *Small Groups: Workable Wineskins*, as a guide in learning about group dynamics. The manual contains information on group sharing, protecting confidentiality in a group, keeping discussion moving, expressing feelings appropriately, listening actively, and dealing with silent times.[6]

Nancy Clodfelder, who had been trained at Pine Rest Christian Hospital in *Amity* listening skills, provided the training in listening (see pp. 118-120). She emphasized that listening is a learned skill requiring practice and, when learned, becomes a caring action. Both Rev. Kretzschmer and Ms. Clodfelder are members of Westminster Presbyterian Church. They volunteered to train the volunteers who would lead the support groups. (We expected our volunteers to have some background in communication skills as well.)

Next we tried to determine the size of the group. Most experts recommended approximately 13 people as the best size group. When we visited an Alcoholics Anonymous support group, we found that they set no limits on the number of people who could attend. We have found that 20 people per session is about the maximum size of a successful group. When more than 20 attend, a new group should be formed. We also found that approximately 1½ hours is a good length for each session.

The next step was to find a room (in a church, hospital, community building, business, or elsewhere) that was large enough to accommodate the group, was comfortable, and would be available for every meeting. We found just the right setting for the support group in one of the conference rooms at Westminster Presbyterian Church. We also charged a small fee to cover costs, which included volunteer expenses, coffee, cookies, name tags, the Myers-Briggs Type Indicator tests, and so forth. A reminder: be sure to order the Myers-Briggs tests at least a month before you need them (address given on p. 145).

We then organized a theme for each meeting. This concept was fashioned after the Alcoholics Anonymous support groups. (Visiting an AA group, with permission, is another tool for training staff.) We organized the themes by looking at the concepts we thought most important in the quitting process. For example, we felt that anger, stress, and self-confidence were important and needed to be understood and controlled by the participant. In addition, we came up with nine other themes for a total of twelve themes. Since the support groups are ongoing, after the twelfth week, we continued the support programs by going back to theme number one, anger.

Weekly meetings

First Week: The theme is *anger*. Each week the staff leaders meet the participants as they arrive, give them name tags, and invite them to sit in chairs arranged in a circle. The meeting is opened with prayer. The discussion is started by introducing the theme. The leaders then suggest concepts such as the facts that smokers use cigarettes to keep a lid on their anger (see Chapter 1) and that when quitting, many people become angry because they have to give up something they like (see Chapter 9). The leaders illustrate these points with personal stories. They further suggest, according to Gary R. Collins in his book *Christian Counseling*, that 80 percent of the anger felt by each of us comes because of the actions of other people. Collins suggests that anger is a reaction of indignation in response to some person or situation.[7] They then ask the group to share how quitting smoking has affected their anger.

At the end of the meeting, the staff might suggest that avoiding anger-arousing situations and people, learning to evaluate situations, building their self-esteem, avoiding ruminating, learning to confront, and stronger self-control might be ways to prevent anger.[8] End with prayer.

Second Week: The theme is *stress*. After prayer and introduction of the theme, the leaders suggest concepts about stress such as "many smokers handle stress by smoking." How do they now handle stress, plus the additional stress generated by a change? (See Chapter 10.) The leaders should illustrate these points with personal stories. They further suggest that, according to Wayne Weiten, the four major sources of psychological stress are *frustration* (you want something you can't have), *conflict* (you have to decide between two goals), *pressure* (expectations to behave in a certain way), and *change* (altered routines).[9] Ask the group to share their frustrations, conflicts, pressures, and changes while quitting.

At the end of the meeting, the staff leaders might read the ways to deal with stress as suggested in Chapter 10. End with prayer.

Third Week: The theme is *visualization—guided imagery.* After prayer and introduction of the theme, the leaders suggest that visualization is a tool or technique to help one quit smoking. It can be used for change and growth by tapping one's inner strength. For example, a person can visualize him- or herself first as a smoker, then as a nonsmoker (see Chapters 7 and 10). The staff leaders should tell their personal stories. They then ask the group to share how they might envision themselves as nonsmokers. You may wish to use guided imagery during the meeting, adapting one of the exercises at the end of Chapter 10 (pp. 93-95).

At the end of the meeting, the leaders should have available for sale a guided image cassette tape for those who wish to use this method to remain a nonsmoker. End with prayer.

Fourth Week: The theme is *learning about your smoker-within.* After prayer and introduction of the theme, the leaders suggest that each participant confront their smoker-within, assuming responsibility and ownership of their smoking habit (see Chapter 6 for responsibility, ownership, process, and related topics). The staff leaders should illustrate these points with personal stories. They then ask the group to share how they confront their smoker-within.

At the end of the meeting, the staff should point out that to quit smoking is a *process.* End with prayer.

Fifth Week: The theme is *meditation: seeking God's help.* After prayer and introduction of the theme, the leaders share that God's power is a loving power that promotes life. The good news is that this power of God's is available for all persons. All we have to do is ask (see Chapter 5). God's power can help us conquer smoking. The staff illustrates this point with a personal story, then asks group participants to share how they individually seek God's help.

At the end of the meeting the leaders suggest that daily prayer is important. They should remind participants that God often works through other people and encourage them to ask friends for help. End with prayer.

Sixth Week: The theme is *goal setting*. After prayer and introduction of the theme, the leaders share that to set goals is the beginning of a commitment—a commitment to change a bad habit. To set goals is the beginning of action toward a better life-style (see Chapter 8). The leaders might share their personal goals and how setting goals moved them toward a better life-style. The leaders then ask the participants to share their goals.

At the end of the meeting, the leaders might read the suggested goals from Chapter 8 (see pp. 72-74). If the participants have not made their own goals, now might be the time to start. End with prayer. (Send home a copy of the Myers-Briggs Type Indicator test with those who will be coming next week.)

Seventh Week: The theme is *Myers-Briggs Type Indicator test*. (Copies of the test may be obtained from Consulting Psychologists Press, Inc., 577 College Ave., Palo Alto, CA 94306.) This test, as previously indicated in Chapter 7, is a tool to help understand individual personality makeup and preferences—that is, whether a person is more highly developed in thinking or feeling, in sensation or functions, is an introvert or an extrovert, and so forth. You probably wonder what all this has to do with giving up smoking. Basically, we believe that many people change their lives while giving up a habit. This means they will be looking at their family life, their work situations, how they play, what organizations they are a part of, their friends, and other important aspects of their lives. It will be very important for them to understand themselves and how they relate to the world in order that wise decisions are made.

For example, Lucy decided to quit smoking. She and her husband Ron were having trouble with their marriage and her question became: Should I divorce Ron? After taking the Myers-Briggs Type Indicator test, Lucy learned that she was an extrovert, or a person who is energized by interaction with others. She asked Ron to take the same test and he learned that he is an introvert, or a person who renews his energy during a period of turning inward and aloneness. Lucy handled her depression by going to a party or shopping. Ron handled his depression by shutting himself away from people. The test gave Lucy a new insight into her relationship with Ron.

Lucy was also having trouble at work with her boss, Sue, who came across as a stern and uncaring person who didn't appreciate Lucy's efforts to do a good job. Lucy's question became: Should I quit my job? The Myers-Briggs Type Indicator test showed that Lucy arrives at many decisions through her own value system, a system that takes one's own self and others into account. This is called a *feeling* function. When Lucy thought about her boss she realized that Sue reaches decisions through a logical process, one of analysis called a *thinking* process. If analysis was not achieved, Sue became critical and stated her position bluntly, often hurting Lucy without knowing it. Lucy was now able to look at her boss in a different light.[10]

Other dimensions of Lucy's personality were uncovered from this test, such as her competitive nature, her super-sensitivity, her need to be stroked, her need to achieve goals, to belong, and so forth.[11]

This test enables stop-smoking instructors to decide how to help certain groups of people deal with their problems. For example, the group of people who score high on the test as introverts, sensing, thinking, and judging, generally like order and routine in their lives. They are more apt to want the help of the support group to help them sort and put their lives back into order. On the other hand, those people who use the intuition function need the support group as a sounding board. They want to share ideas on how to change. We have found the Myers-Briggs Type Indicator test very helpful in interpreting how people change.

After prayer and introduction of the theme, the leaders share how the Myers-Briggs Type Indicator test helped them discover various aspects of their own personality and how it helped them understand other people's personalities. The group then shares some of their results. (We recommend that a volunteer, trained in the Myers-Briggs Type Indicator test, be asked to explain the results of the test to participants.) End the meeting with prayer.

Eighth Week: The theme is *sabotage: lapse/relapse*. After prayer and introduction of the theme, the leaders suggest that sabotage is the deliberate attempt by your smoker-within to smoke. The leaders might share the story of Lou and her little con in Chapter 12 (see pp. 102-103). Share how people trying to quit smoking have a little con sitting on their shoulders shouting for them to smoke. The leaders then illustrate these points with a personal story. Then the leaders ask the group to share their stories of sabotage (see Chapter 12).

Toward the end of the meeting, use the puppet show (see pp. 150-152) or some related activity, perhaps personal stories or dialogs about inner conflict. Close with prayer.

Ninth Week: The theme is *adjusting to loss: the grief process*. After prayer and introduction of the theme, the leaders might suggest that when one quits smoking, one loses a good friend. Because of this loss, one will experience various stages of grief. The leaders might list the stages of the grief process suggested by Elisabeth Kübler-Ross (see Chapter 9), on a chalkboard. Then illustrate the stages with personal stories. The leaders then ask the group to think about their loss and the various stages. (This might be the time to ask the doctor or psychologist on the stop-smoking board to explain depression and ways to handle depression.) End the meeting with prayer.

Tenth Week: The theme is *building new self-confidence*. After prayer and introduction of the theme, the leaders suggest that the image we have of ourselves determines our life-style and our feelings of worth. The way we see ourselves—strong, weak, good-looking, homely, friendly, or whatever—determines the image we have of ourselves. What we often forget, however, is that all people have both strengths and weaknesses. What we must remember is that those with strong self-confidence work on their strengths instead of dwelling on their weaknesses (see Chapter 7). The leaders might illustrate these points with personal stories. Then ask the group to talk about their self-image and how they might build more self-confidence.

At the end of the meeting, share the four techniques given in Chapter 7 on how to develop a stronger self-confidence. End with prayer.

Eleventh Week: The theme is *trust vs. fear*. After prayer and introduction of the theme, the leaders suggest that trusting oneself to be a successful nonsmoker gives freedom. Fear, on the other hand, constrains and blocks and takes away freedom. If instead of trust there is fear, quitting smoking will not be successful. The leaders might illustrate these points with personal stories. They ask the group to share their feelings on trust and fear.

End the meeting by emphasizing that trusting in the Lord and asking for the Lord's power can help us defeat fear. End with prayer.

Twelfth Week: The theme is *altering your regular behavior patterns*. After prayer and introduction of the theme, the leaders suggest that changing personal patterns and rituals that support the smoking habit is a "must" if one is to quit smoking. Begin by changing actions in your "public world." After some time, changes will begin to take place in your "private world." In other words, actions are the beginning of changed attitudes. The leaders might use personal stories to illustrate the point. Then ask all members of the group to share how they might alter their behavior patterns (see Chapter 5). End the meeting with prayer.

On the thirteenth week, begin a new 12-week cycle by using the first theme again. Support is an important key in becoming a successful nonsmoker. If an ongoing support system such as the one just described here is not available, find a friend, another Christian, or a family member to support your efforts.

Join an Alcoholics Anonymous support group

The Alcoholics Anonymous (AA) Twelve Step Plan[12] may be adapted for new nonsmokers as a support system.

Many people who have gone through our retreats and/or clinics have gone on to work through the twelve steps as a vital means of support to see them through the stop-smoking process. Ruth Mysliwiec, a volunteer in our program, has adapted these steps for new nonsmokers:

1. We admitted we were powerless over nicotine—that our lives had become unmanageable.
2. Came to believe that a Power greater than ourselves could restore us to sanity.
3. Made a decision to turn our will and our lives over to the care of God as we understood God.
4. Made a searching and fearless moral inventory of ourselves.
5. Admitted to God, to ourselves, and to another human being the exact nature of our wrongs.
6. Were entirely ready to have God remove all these defects of character.
7. Humbly asked God to remove our shortcomings.
8. Made a list of all persons we had harmed, and became willing to make amends to them all.
9. Made direct amends to such people whenever possible, except when to do so would injure them or others.
10. Continued to take personal inventory, and when we were wrong, promptly admitted it.
11. Sought through prayer and meditation to improve our conscious contact with God as we understood God, praying only for knowledge of God's will for us and the power to carry that out.
12. Having had a spiritual awakening as the result of these steps, we tried to carry this message to addicts, and to practice these principles in all our affairs.

Puppet show

Nancy Clodfelder created a puppet show that uses two puppets to demonstrate the battle that goes on between a person's two forces—the smoker-within and the nonsmoker-within. In our program we constantly work to help the nonsmoker-within to become stronger than the smoker. When this finally occurs, the smoker will become a nonsmoker.

As you design your own stop-smoking program, you may wish to incorporate the puppet show into your program. It may be used at any time. The conversation follows here:

SMOKER: Wow, I don't know what I'm going to do now. I just ate supper and am about to go nuts wanting a cigarette. I know that I shouldn't, but I really need it or I'll go crazy.

NONSMOKER: Hey there, it sounds to me like you are really having a hard time. It sounds like you're feeling very nervous about this.

SMOKER: Oh, you don't know anything. I've always smoked and you *know* how much I enjoy it.

NONSMOKER: Yes, I know that you enjoy it and you think that you won't be able to enjoy anything without having a cigarette.

SMOKER: Yes, my nerves are jittery, my stomach hurts, and I can't seem to remember anything.

NONSMOKER: You really *are* a wreck, but do you remember what they told us at the class about this?

SMOKER: Oh, come off it. I don't want to hear about the class. I'm sick of hearing about the class. Everyone knows that I'm there, and that's embarrassing because they think I probably won't make it.

NONSMOKER: Say, I wonder if now isn't the time to look at *you*, Smoker, and not your peers. *You* are the one that is fighting this, not your friends. Maybe they're saying these things to make you a little nervous about all of this. I'm a little uneasy myself but I want to win. I desire it, want it, wish for it, and prefer not to smoke. You're self-destructive and negative about everything. You're so demanding and commanding and insistent. You're hard to beat. I'm trying to be nice to you because I know that you're suffering. You've been a part of me for a long time and I thought of you as a real friend. Seeing you in such stress is like having a part of *me* so tense. I want to help you. But, I also want clean lungs, relaxation, recreation, a seat in the nonsmoking section, to run again, to smell again, to take a deep breath, to see a lot of tomorrows. . . .

SMOKER: Well, Nonsmoker, you have a good argument. I'll try not to be such a pest in your new outlook. I know that you want to win. You're a part of me. Maybe it's your turn to be in charge of our life together. I know that this way, the chances for us to live longer are very real. I also know that I like you and you care about us. You are a very real friend to me now. I respect you for trying to win this battle for us. Thanks for listening to me, my friend. I'm tired now after our talk. You won this time, you ole nonsmoker-within. I'm not licked yet, but keep up the good work and we'll both come out winners!

Sample Evaluation Form

Date _____

Stop-smoking Services

Evaluation

1. In what ways do you feel you benefited from this program?

2. What adjustments could be made in the program to improve it?

3. Would you consider recommending this program to a friend? Why or why not?

4. Was the time during which the program was offered convenient for you? If not, what would be a better time?

5. Please provide specific comments on the program content and the instructors.

6. Is there anything else we should know?

7. How did you hear about this seminar?

Thank you for your input. With your help, we hope to achieve high quality and effectiveness and better serve your needs and interests.

Sample Application Form

Stop-smoking Services

Sponsored by Westminster–Eastminster Presbyterian
Churches
Grand Rapids, Michigan

Name_____ Date_____
Address_____ Home phone_____
City_____ ZIP_____ Business phone_____
Tuition fee_____ Deposit with application_____
(Make check payable to Westminster Presbyterian
Church, 47 Jefferson S.E., Grand Rapids, MI 49503.)

Please provide the information requested. If you need
more space, use the back of the paper.

History

Age_____Sex_____Height_____Weight_____
Place of birth_____
Environment during childhood and adolescence:
Rural____Small town____Suburban____Urban_____
Environment during adult life:
Rural____Small town____Suburban____Urban_____

Present occupation_____No. of years_____
Previous occupation_____No. of years_____

Medical history

Illnesses:

Personal history of allergy:
Asthma_____ Hay Fever_____ Hives_____ Eczema_____

Family history of smoking

Father: Smoker_____Duration of habit _____
       Cigarette_____Cigar_____Pipe_____
Mother: Smoker_____Duration of habit _____
       Cigarette_____Cigar_____Pipe_____

If either is deceased, please state cause:

List brothers and sisters and state whether they are smokers and at what age they started smoking:

Family history of allergy

Does any close relative have asthma, hay fever, hives, or eczema? Please list relationship to you and disease:

Personal smoking history

Age started _____Years smoked _____Packs per day_____

Cigarette_____Cigar_____ Pipe_____

List previous attempts to stop-smoking:
What year_____Duration of attempt _____
Reason for resuming _____

List reasons you originally started smoking:

Did you enjoy your first cigarette?

How long did you smoke before it became a pleasurable experience?

Who introduced you to cigarettes, initially?

List reasons you desire to discontinue smoking:

Notes

Chapter 3

1. Gary R. Collins. *Christian Counseling* (Waco, Tex.: Word Books, 1980), pp. 116-127.
2. Alan Loy McGinnis. *Confidence: How to Succeed at Being Yourself* (Minneapolis, Minn.: Augsburg Publishing House, 1987), p. 13.
3. David G. Myers. *Psychology* (New York: Worth Publishers, Inc., 1989).
4. David G. Myers. *Social Psychology* (New York: McGraw-Hill Book Company, 1987), p. 108.
5. David G. Myers. *Psychology* (New York: Worth Publishers, Inc., 1989).
6. David G. Myers. *Social Psychology* (New York: McGraw-Hill Book Company, 1987), p. 105.

Chapter 4

1. Peter Nowell. "The Clonal Evolution of Tumor Cell Population." *Science* 194:23, 1976.
2. U.S. Department of Health and Human Services. "The Health Consequences of Smoking: Cancer—A Report of the Surgeon General." DHHS Publication no. (PHS) 82-50179:9, 1982.
3. Thomas Snick. "Seeking the Possible in Prevention." *ACP Observer* 5:1, 1985.

4. Ibid., p. 14.
5. For this thought we are indebted to David G. Myers, psychology professor at Hope College in Holland, Michigan.
6. R. Levy. "Review: Declining Mortality in Coronary Heart Disease." *Arteriosclerosis* 1:312, 1981.
7. U.S. Department of Health and Human Services. "The Health Consequences of Smoking: Cancer and Chronic Lung Disease in the Workplace—A Report of the Surgeon General." DHHS Publication no. (PHS) 85-50207:33, 1985.
8. Edwin Silverburg and John Lubera. "Cancer Statistics, 1986." *Ca-A Cancer Journal for Clinicians* 36:17, 1986.
9. Ibid., p. 17.
10. Ernest Wynder. "Etiology of Lung Cancer." *Cancer* 30:1332, 1972.
11. Ernest Wynder and Deitrick Hoffman. "Tobacco and Tobacco Smoke." *Seminars in Oncology* 3:5, 1976.
12. Christopher Squier. "Smokeless Tobacco and Oral Cancer: A Cause for Concern?" *Ca-A Cancer Journal for Clinicians* 34:242, 1984.
13. Lynn Rosenberg and David Kaufman, et al. "The Risk of Myocardial Infarction After Quitting Smoking in Men Under 55 Years of Age." *New England Journal of Medicine* 313:1511, 1985.
14. Walter Brueggemann. *Genesis: A Bible Commentary for Teaching and Preaching* (Atlanta, Ga.: John Knox Press, 1982), p. 33.

Chapter 7

1. Alan Loy McGinnis. *Confidence: How to Succeed at Being Yourself* (Minneapolis, Minn.: Augsburg Publishing House, 1987).
2. Ibid., p. 28.
3. This idea used with permission by Dr. Wayne Joosse, Calvin College.

Chapter 8

1. Wayne Weiten, in his book *Psychology Applied to Modern Life: Adjustment in the 80s*, (Monterey, Calif.: Brooks/Cole Publ. Co., 1983), suggests a token economy for reinforcing desired behavior.
2. Morton T. Kelsey. *Adventure Inward* (Minneapolis, Minn.: Augsburg Publishing House, 1980), pp. 23-24. Kelsey encourages the use of journal keeping as a method of handling depression and emotional problems.

3. Ibid., p. 25.
4. Ibid., p. 38.

Chapter 9

1. Material adapted from pp. 38-137 of *On Death and Dying* by Elisabeth Kübler-Ross, copyright © 1969 by Elisabeth Kübler-Ross, is reprinted with permission of Collier Books, an imprint of MacMillan Publishing Co.

Chapter 10

1. O. Carl Simonton, M.D., Stephanie Matthews-Simonton, James L. Creighton. *Getting Well Again* (New York: Bantam Books, Inc., 1978).

Chapter 11

1. David G. Myers. *Psychology* (New York: Worth Publishers, Inc., 1989).
2. Ibid.

Chapter 12

1. Suggested by Alexander Callaghan, professor of Spanish at Grand Rapids Junior College in Grand Rapids, Michigan.
2. U.S. Department of Agriculture and Health and Human Services statistics cited in *The Internist* XXV:6, July 1984, p. 9, in a box titled, "Some Facts about . . . Cigarette Advertising."
3. Matthews L. Myers, "A Smoke-Free Society: An Essential Goal," *The Internist*, July 1984, p. 15.

Appendix

1. Richard P. Walter. *Amity: Friendship in Action* (Kentwood, Mich.: C.H.I., 1980), pp. 18, 22.
2. Ibid., p. 18.
3. These four guidelines are adapted from Wayne Weiten, *Psychology Applied to Modern Life: Adjustment in the 80s* (Monterey, Calif.: Brooks/Cole Publ. Co., 1983), pp. 221-222, with permission.
4. "Why People Smoke Cigarettes," Department of Health and Human Services, p. 1.

5. David G. Myers. *The Human Puzzle* (San Francisco: Harper & Row, 1978), p. 149.

6. Bob Parker. *Small Groups: Workable Wineskins* (Cincinnati, Ohio: Christian Information Committee, 1988), p. 20.

7. Gary R. Collins, *Christian Counseling* (Waco, Tex.: Word Books, 1980), p. 104.

8. Ibid., pp. 112-113.

9. These four sources of psychological stress are adapted from Wayne Weiten, *Psychology Applied to Modern Life: Adjustment in the 80s* (Monterey, Calif.: Brooks/Cole Publ. Co., 1983), pp. 74-79, with permission.

10. These concepts are adapted from Morton T. Kelsey, *Christo-Psychology* (New York: Crossroad Publishing Company, 1982), pp. 68-89.

11. These concepts were suggested by Gary Sweeten, College Hill Presbyterian Church, Cincinnati, Ohio.

12. The Twelve Steps reprinted here in their original wording are adapted with the permission of Alcoholics Anonymous World Services, Inc.: 1) We admitted we were powerless over alcohol—that our lives had become unmanageable. 2) Came to believe that a Power greater than ourselves could restore us to sanity. 3) Made a decision to turn our will and our lives over to the care of God *as we understood Him.* 4) Made a searching and fearless moral inventory of ourselves. 5) Admitted to God, to ourselves, and to another human being the exact nature of our wrongs. 6) Were entirely ready to have God remove all these defects of character. 7) Humbly asked Him to remove our shortcomings. 8) Made a list of all persons we had harmed, and became willing to make amends to them all. 9) Made direct amends to such people wherever possible, except when to do so would injure them or others. 10) Continued to take personal inventory and when we were wrong, promptly admitted it. 11) Sought through prayer and meditation to improve our conscious contact with God *as we understood Him,* praying only for knowledge of His will for us and the power to carry that out. 12) Having had a spiritual awakening as a result of these steps, we tried to carry this message to alcoholics, and to practice these principles in all our affairs.